RENAL
DIET COOKBOOK

*350+ Low-Sodium, Low-Potassium,
Most Tasty And Delicious Recipes To Avoid Dialysis
And Manage Your Kidney Disease*

RENAL DIET COOKBOOK

Copyright 2021 - All rights reserved.

The content contained within this book may not be reproduced, duplicated or transmitted without direct written permission from the author or the publisher.

Under no circumstances will any blame or legal responsibility be held against the publisher, or author, for any damages, reparation, or monetary loss due to the information contained within this book. Either directly or indirectly.

Legal Notice:

This book is copyright protected. This book is only for personal use. You cannot amend, distribute, sell, use, quote or paraphrase any part, or the content within this book, without the consent of the author or publisher.

Disclaimer Notice:

Please note the information contained within this document is for educational and entertainment purposes only. All effort has been executed to present accurate, up to date, and reliable, complete information. No warranties of any kind are declared or implied. Readers acknowledge that the author is not engaging in the rendering of legal, financial, medical or professional advice. The content within this book has been derived from various sources. Please consult a licensed professional before attempting any techniques outlined in this book.

By reading this document, the reader agrees that under no circumstances is the author responsible for any losses, direct or indirect, which are incurred as a result of the use of information contained within this document, including, but not limited to, errors, omissions, or inaccuracies.

RENAL DIET COOKBOOK

Table of Contents

INTRODUCTION 10

CHAPTER 1: THE KIDNEY DISEASE 12
- WHAT IS KIDNEY DISEASE? 12
- EPIDEMIOLOGY - CHRONIC KIDNEY DISEASE: CLASSIFICATION, RISK FACTORS, AND HISTORY 12
- WHO RUNS THE RISK OF HAVING A CKD? 13

CHAPTER 2: WHAT YOU CAN EAT AND WHAT YOU SHOULD AVOID IN RENAL DIET 16
- FOODS TO EAT 16
- FOODS TO AVOID 17
- FLUIDS AND JUICES FOR HEALTHY KIDNEYS 17

CHAPTER 3: BREAKFAST 18
1. Berry Chia with Yogurt 18
2. Arugula Eggs with Chili Peppers 18
3. Breakfast Skillet 18
4. Eggplant Chicken Sandwich 19
5. Panzanella Salad 20
6. Shrimp Bruschetta 20
7. Strawberry Muesli 21
8. Yogurt Bulgur 21
9. Chia Pudding 21
10. Yufka Pies 22
11. Egg White Scramble 22
12. Beet Smoothie 22
13. Chia Bars 23
14. Pineapple Smoothie 23
15. Cauliflower Rice and Coconut 23
16. Kale and Garlic Platter 24
17. Lemon and Broccoli Platter 24
18. Garlic and Butter-Flavored Cod 24
19. Egg White and Pepper Omelet 25
20. Italian Apple Fritters 25
21. Tofu and Mushroom Scramble 26
22. Egg Fried Rice 26
23. Quick Thai Chicken and Vegetable Curry 27
24. Cajun Stuffed Peppers 27
25. Stuffed Zucchini 28
26. Savory Collard Chips 28
27. Blackberry Pudding 29
28. Simple Green Shake 29
29. Fine Morning Porridge 29
30. Hungarian's Porridge 30
31. Zucchini and Onion Platter 30
32. Collard Greens Dish 30
33. Simple Zucchini BBQ 31
34. Angel Eggs 31
35. Denver Omelets 32
36. Scrambled Eggs and Pesto 32
37. Lemon Broccoli 32
38. Eggplant Fries 33
39. Pineapple Oatmeal 33
40. Simple Chia Porridge 33
41. Pepperoni Omelet 34
42. Scrambled Turkey Eggs 34
43. Cinnamon Flavored Baked Apple Chips 34
44. Apple & Cinnamon French Toast 35
45. Blueberry Smoothie in a Bowl 35
46. Egg Pockets 36
47. Italian Eggs with Peppers 36
48. Mushroom Omelet 37
49. Asparagus Frittata 37
50. Poached Eggs with Cilantro Butter 38
51. Chorizo and Egg Tortilla 39
52. Cottage Pancakes 39
53. Egg in a Hole 40
54. German Pancakes 40
55. Mushroom and Red Pepper Omelet 41
56. Apple and Zucchini Bread 41
57. Spicy Corn Bread 42
58. Breakfast Casserole 43
59. Cauliflower Tortilla 43
60. Eggs Benedict 44
61. Cranberry and Apple Oatmeal 45
62. Blueberry Breakfast Smoothie 45
63. Apple Sauce Cream Toast 46
64. Waffles 46
65. Egg Whites and Veggie Bake 47
66. Peach Berry Parfait 48
67. Open-Faced Bagel Breakfast Sandwich 48
68. Bulgur Bowl with Strawberries and Walnuts 49
69. Overnight Oats Three Ways 49
70. Buckwheat Pancakes 50
71. Broccoli Basil Quiche 51
72. Poor Knight with Apple Compote 51

73. Papaya and Cranberry Jam 52
74. Lemon Curd 52
75. Pancakes with Raspberries and Ricotta 53
76. Muesli Made From Rice Flakes 53
77. Muesli Mix 53
78. Bamboo Bread (Low Carb) 54
79. Open Bread with Avocado 54
80. Bircher Muesli with Papaya 54
81. Cauliflower and Broccoli Curry 55
82. Broccoli and Lentil Salad with Mackerel 55
83. Broccoli Rice Gratin (Italian Style) 56
84. Colorful Bean Salad 57

CHAPTER 4: MAIN DISHES 58

85. Corn and Shrimp Quiche 58
86. Ginger-Orange Tuna Pasta Salad 58
87. Pineapple-Soy Salmon Stir-Fry 59
88. Fish Taco Filling 60
89. Ginger Shrimp with Snow Peas 60
90. Roasted Cod with Plums 61
91. Lemon Chicken 61
92. Curried Chicken Stir-Fry 62
93. Thai-Style Chicken Salad 63
94. Chicken Casserole 63
95. Chicken Patties with Dill 64
96. Chicken and Cabbage Stir-Fry 65
97. Slow Cooker Chicken with Apple and Onions . 66
98. Herbed Chicken and Veggies 66
99. Aussie Turkey 67
100. Coriander Chicken with Pineapple Salsa 67
101. Honey Chicken Kabobs 68
102. Chicken Scampi 69
103. Chicken with Quinoa and Wild Rice 69
104. Pineapple and Mint Lamb Chops 70
105. Maple-Brined Pork Loin 70
106. Beef Stir-Fry 71
107. Pork Picadillo 72
108. Beef Bulgogi 72
109. Creamy Chicken with Cider 73
110. Exotic Palabok 73
111. Vegetarian Gobi Curry 74
112. Marinated Shrimp and Pasta 74
113. Steak and Onion Sandwich 75
114. Zesty Crab Cakes 75
115. Tofu Hoisin Sauté 76
116. Zucchini Noodles with Spring Vegetables ... 77
117. Stir-Fried Vegetables 77
118. Lime Asparagus Spaghetti 78
119. Garden Crustless Quiche 78
120. Lentil Veggie Burgers 79
121. Baked Cauliflower Rice Cakes 80
122. Marinated Paprika Chicken 80
123. Cool Cucumber Salad 81
124. Sautéed Butternut Squash 81
125. Herb Roasted Chicken 81
126. Seared Scallops 82
127. Dolmas Wrap 82
128. Salad al Tonno 83
129. Arlecchino Rice Salad 83
130. Greek Salad 84
131. Baked Vegetables Soup 84
132. Pesto Chicken Salad 84
133. Falafel 85
134. Israeli Pasta Salad 86
135. Artichoke Matzo Mina 86
136. Sautéed Chickpea and Lentil Mix 87
137. Buffalo Chicken Lettuce Wraps 87
138. Crazy Japanese Potato and Beef Croquettes 88
139. Spicy Chili Crackers 88
140. Golden Eggplant Fries 89
141. Traditional Black Bean Chili 89
142. Very Wild Mushroom Pilaf 89
143. Green Palak Paneer 90

CHAPTER 5: FISH AND SEAFOOD 92

144. Shrimp Paella 92
145. Salmon and Pesto Salad 92
146. Baked Fennel and Garlic Sea Bass 93
147. Lemon, Garlic & Cilantro Tuna and Rice 93
148. Cod & Green Bean Risotto 94
149. Mixed Pepper Stuffed River Trout 94
150. Haddock & Buttered Leeks 95
151. Thai Spiced Halibut 95
152. Monk-Fish Curry 96
153. Oregon Tuna Patties 96
154. Fish Chowder 97
155. Broiled Sesame Cod 97
156. Tuna Salad with Cranberries 98
157. Zucchini Cups with Dill Cream and Smoked Tuna 98
158. Creamy Smoked Tuna Macaroni 99
159. Asparagus and Smoked Tuna Salad 99
160. Spicy Tuna Salad Sandwiches 100
161. Spanish Tuna 100

162. Fish with Vegetables 101
163. Creamy Crab over Salmon 101
164. Fish Tacos 102
165. Jambalaya 103
166. Asparagus Shrimp Linguini 103
167. Tuna Noodle Casserole 104
168. Oven-Fried Southern Style Catfish 105
169. Cilantro-Lime Cod 106
170. Shrimp Quesadilla 106

CHAPTER 6: MEAT 108

171. Pork Souvlaki 108
172. Open-Faced Beef Stir-Up 108
173. Grilled Steak with Cucumber Salsa 109
174. Beef Brisket 109
175. Lamb Shoulder with Zucchini and Eggplant
.... 110
176. Beef Chili 110
177. Skirt Steak Glazed with Bourbon 111
178. Beef Pot Roast 112
179. Grilled Lamb Chops 112
180. Lamb & Pineapple Kebabs 112
181. Baked Meatballs & Scallions 113
182. Pork with Bell Pepper 114
183. Pork with Pineapple 115
184. Pork Chili 116
185. Ground Pork with Water Chestnuts 116
186. Hearty Meatloaf 117
187. Chicken with Mushrooms 118

CHAPTER 7: POULTRY 120

188. Roasted Citrus Chicken 120
189. Chicken with Asian Vegetables 120
190. Chicken Adobo 121
191. Chicken and Veggie Soup 121
192. Turkey Sausages 122
193. Smoky Turkey Chili 122
194. Rosemary Chicken 123
195. Herbs and Lemony Roasted Chicken 123
196. Ground Chicken & Peas Curry 124
197. Chicken Meatballs Curry 124

CHAPTER 8: SOUP 126

198. Chicken and Corn Soup 126
199. Pumpkin Bacon Soup 126
200. Classic Chicken Soup 127
201. Beef Okra Soup 127
202. Chicken Pasta Soup 128
203. Cream of Watercress Soup 128
204. Curried Cauliflower Soup 129
205. Asparagus Lemon Soup 129

CHAPTER 9: SALAD 132

206. Hawaiian Chicken Salad 132
207. Grated Carrot Salad with Lemon-Dijon
Vinaigrette 132
208. Tuna Macaroni Salad 133
209. Couscous Salad 133
210. Fruity Zucchini Salad 133
211. Cucumber Salad, Pulled Through Slowly . 134
212. Tortellini Salad 134
213. Farmer's Salad 135
214. Chicken and Asparagus Salad with
Watercress 135
215. Cucumber Salad 136
216. Thai Cucumber Salad 136
217. Broccoli-Cauliflower Salad 137
218. Macaroni Salad 137

CHAPTER 10: SOUP, SALAD, SNACKS & LIGHT MEALS RECIPES 138

219. Cinnamon Apple Chips 138
220. Roasted Red Pepper Hummus 138
221. Thai-Style Eggplant Dip 139
222. Collard Salad Rolls with Peanut Dipping
Sauce 139
223. Simple Roasted Broccoli 140
224. Roasted Mint Carrots 140
225. Roasted Root Vegetables 141
226. Vegetable Couscous 141
227. Garlic Cauliflower Rice 142
228. Creamy Broccoli Soup 142
229. Curried Carrot and Beet Soup 143
230. Golden Beet Soup 143
231. Cauliflower and Chive Soup 144
232. Salad with Vinaigrette 145
233. Salad with Lemon Dressing 145
234. Shrimp with Salsa 145
235. Cauliflower Soup 146
236. Cabbage Stew 147
237. Eggplant and Red Pepper Soup 147
238. Kale Chips 148
239. Tortilla Chips 148
240. Corn Bread 149

241. Vegetable Rolls 149
242. Frittata with Penne 150
243. Tofu Stir-Fry 150
244. Cauliflower Patties 151
245. Turnip Chips 151
246. Chicken and Mandarin Salad 152
247. Roasted Red Pepper Soup 152
248. Leek and Carrot Soup 152
249. Creamy Vinaigrette 153
250. Chicken and Pasta Salad 153
251. Herbed Soup with Black Beans 154
252. Creamy Pumpkin Soup 154
253. Lemony Lentil Salad with Salmon 155
254. Spaghetti Squash & Yellow Bell-Pepper Soup 155
255. Red Pepper & Brie Soup 156
256. Turkey & Lemon-Grass Soup 156
257. Paprika Pork Soup 157
258. Mediterranean Vegetable Soup 157
259. Tofu Soup 158
260. Onion Soup 158
261. Steakhouse Soup 159
262. Pear & Brie Salad 159
263. Caesar Salad 159

CHAPTER 11: SPICE BLENDS AND SEASONING... 162

264. Creole Seasoning Mix 162
265. Adobo Seasoning Mix 162
266. Lamb and Pork Seasoning 163
267. Asian Seasoning 163
268. Onion Seasoning Blend 163
269. Apple Pie Spice 164
270. Poultry Seasoning 164
271. Hot Curry Powder 165
272. Cajun Seasoning 165
273. Berbere spice mix 165

CHAPTER 12: VEGETABLES 168

274. Thai Tofu Broth 168
275. Delicious Vegetarian Lasagna 168
276. Chili Tofu Noodles 169
277. Curried Cauliflower 170
278. Chinese Tempeh Stir Fry 170
279. Egg White Frittata with Penne 170
280. Vegetable Fried Rice 171
281. Vegetable Biryani 172
282. Couscous Burgers 172

283. Marinated Tofu Stir-Fry 173
284. Curried Veggie Stir-Fry 173
285. Chilaquiles 174
286. Roasted Veggie Sandwiches 175
287. Pasta Fagioli 176
288. Roasted Peach Open-Face Sandwich .. 177
289. Spicy Corn and Rice Burritos 177
290. Crustless Cabbage Quiche 178
291. Vegetable Confetti Relish 179
292. Creamy Veggie Casserole 179
293. Vegetable Green Curry 180
294. Zucchini Bowl 180
295. Nice Coconut Haddock 181
296. Vegetable Rice Casserole 181

CHAPTER 13: SMOOTHIES AND DRINKS 184

297. Almonds & Blueberries Smoothie 184
298. Almonds and Zucchini Smoothie 184
299. Blueberries and Coconut Smoothie 185
300. Collard Greens and Cucumber Smoothie ... 185
301. Creamy Dandelion Greens and Celery Smoothie 186
302. Dark Turnip Greens Smoothie 186
303. Butter Pecan and Coconut Smoothie .. 187
304. Fresh Cucumber, Kale, and Raspberry Smoothie 187
305. Green Coconut Smoothie 188
306. Fresh Lettuce and Cucumber-Lemon Smoothie 188
307. Instant Coffee Smoothie 189
308. Keto Blood Sugar Adjuster Smoothie ... 189
309. Lime Smoothie 190
310. Protein Coconut Smoothie 190
311. Total Almond Smoothie 191
312. Ultimate Green Mix Smoothie 191
313. Hot Cocoa 192
314. Cinnamon and Hazelnut Coffee 192
315. Almond Milk 193
316. Cucumber and Lemon-Flavored Water 193

CHAPTER 14: SNACKS 194

317. Sesame-Garlic Edamame 194
318. Rosemary and White Bean Dip 194
319. Garlicky Cale Chips 195
320. Baked Tortilla Chips 195
321. Spicy Guacamole 196
322. Chickpea Fatteh 196

323. Marinated Berries 197
324. Pumpkin-Turmeric Latte 197
325. Dark Hot Chocolate 197
326. Dark Chocolate and Cherry Trail Mix 198
327. Happy Heart Energy Bites......................... 198
328. Chocolate-Cashew Spread 199
329. Mango Chiller 199
330. Blueberry-Ricotta Swirl 200
331. Roasted Broccoli and Cauliflower 200
332. Herbed Garlic Cauliflower Mash............. 200
333. Sautéed Spicy Cabbage 201
334. Fragrant Thai-Style Eggplant................... 201
335. Roasted Asparagus with Pine Nuts 202
336. Roasted Radishes 202
337. Grilled Peppers in Chipotle Vinaigrette 203
338. Double Corn Muffins 203

CHAPTER 15: DESSERTS 206

339. Spiced Peaches 206
340. Pumpkin Cheesecake Bar 206
341. Blueberry Mini Muffins 207
342. Baked Peaches with Cream Cheese 207
343. Bread Pudding... 208
344. Strawberry Ice Cream 209
345. Cinnamon Custard 209
346. Raspberry Brule....................................... 210
347. Tart Apple Granita 210
348. Lemon-Lime Sherbet 211
349. Pavlova with Peaches 211
350. Tropical Vanilla Snow Cone 212
351. Rhubarb Crumble 213
352. Gingerbread Loaf 213
353. Elegant Lavender Cookies....................... 214
354. Carob Angel Food Cake 214
355. Old-fashioned Apple Kuchen 215
356. Dessert Cocktail 216
357. Baked Egg Custard 216
358. Gumdrop Cookies 216
359. Pound Cake with Pineapple 217
360. Apple Crunch Pie..................................... 217
361. Vanilla Custard.. 218
362. Chocolate Chip Cookies 218
363. Coconut Loaf 219
364. Chocolate Parfait 219
365. Cauliflower Bagel.................................... 220
366. Lemon Mousse... 220
367. Jalapeno Crisp 220
368. Raspberry Popsicle.................................. 221
369. Easy Fudge.. 221
370. Cashew and Almond Butter..................... 222
371. Instant Pot Cheesecake.......................... 222
372. Pots De Crème 223
373. Ingredient Cheesecake........................... 223
374. Egg Leche Flan.. 224
375. Pot Chocolate Pudding Cake 225
376. Carrot Cake 225
377. Pumpkin Chocolate Cake........................ 226
378. Apple Pie 226
379. Blueberry Cream Cones 227
380. Cherry Coffee Cake 227
381. Cherry Dessert 228
382. Crunchy Peppermint Cookies.................. 228
383. Cranberries Snow.................................... 229
384. Chia Pudding with Berries....................... 230
385. Vanilla Delight... 230
386. Chocolate Beet Cake.............................. 230
387. Strawberry Pie 231
388. Grape Skillet Galette 232
389. Small Chocolate Cakes 232
390. Strawberry Whipped Cream Cake 233
391. Sweet Cracker Pie Crust 233
392. Apple Oatmeal Crunchy 234
393. Berry Ice Cream 234
394. Deliciously Good Scones........................ 234
395. Mixed Berry Cobbler............................... 235
396. Blueberry Espresso Brownies.................. 235
397. Coffee Brownies 236
398. Keto Marshmellow 236

CONCLUSION......................................238

Introduction

The kidneys are two incredibly powerful organs. When a person has two healthy and fully functioning kidneys, these organs can filter four ounces of blood, removing waste and impurities from it every minute. During the process of filtering this blood, not only do the kidneys remove waste, but they also remove a little excess fluid to create urine and remove the waste. After this process, the waste-filled fluid is pushed to the bladder, where it will become urine before being expelled from the body.

You can do many things if you want to keep your kidneys healthy and have them functioning properly. Here are certain instructions that you can keep in mind for ensuring the proper functioning of your kidneys.

You should always make certain that you are sufficiently hydrated, but you shouldn't overdo this. No studies have shown that over-hydration is good for enhancing the performance of your kidneys. It is good to drink sufficient water and drink around four to six water glasses per day. Consuming more water than this wouldn't help your kidneys perform better. It would just increase the stress on your kidneys.

Your kidneys are capable of tolerating a wide variety of dietary habits. Usually, most kidney problems crop up from other existing medical conditions, like high blood pressure or diabetes. Thus, it would be advisable to consume foods that will help you regulate your weight and blood pressure. If you were able to prevent diabetes and even high blood pressure, then your kidneys would be healthy as well.

If you were already consuming healthy foods, it would also make sense if you were exercising regularly because regular physical activity will prevent weight gain and also regulate your blood pressure. But you should be careful about the amount of time you exercise or how much you exercise, especially if you aren't acclimatized to exercising. Don't overexert yourself if you are just getting started because this would increase the pressure on your kidneys and result in the breaking down of your muscles.

Since the kidneys filter the blood, people may mistakenly believe that the kidneys are like a sponge that absorbs and hold onto any waste or impurities. However, this is not true. The kidneys may remove waste and toxins from the blood, but rather than holding onto it; they have a process to eliminate it in our system.

Kidney failure has no treatment to reverse it, and it is essential to take a truly healthy diet that protects your body from any kind of health hazards associated with kidney disease. However, if you suffer from kidney failure or any other kidney disease, there is no reason to give up hope; with proper treatment and diet, the management you can live a healthy and long life.

You have to start producing healthy lifestyle choices, and it begins with healthy changes to your diet. The news is that once you start your kidney treatment and maintain your ideal diet, its associated symptoms start to go away.

Good dietary habits are known to keep kidney diseases at bay. It's time to make smart choices when it comes to food that you eat every day. An ideal renal diet is all about including wholesome foods and reducing the number of products, which contain high sodium, high phosphorous, and high potassium.

An ideal renal diet restricts foods that are harmful to your kidney and renal system. This exclusive book on a renal diet is based on recipes that reduce the consumption of sodium, phosphorous, potassium and provide your body with healthy nutrients to avoid unwanted health symptoms and complications.

Explore the collection of healthy, homemade recipes for chronic kidney diseases. The purpose of recipes is to avoid stress to your kidneys without compromising on taste value. This represents delicious and flavorful recipes, including breakfast, salads, soups, stews, chicken and poultry mains, meat mains, fish and seafood mains, vegetarian mains, and desserts.

CHAPTER 1:

The Kidney Disease

What is Kidney Disease?

There is chronic kidney disease (CKD) when damaged kidneys or kidney function decline for three months or more. There are five stages of evolution of a CRM according to the severity of the renal involvement or the degree of deterioration of its function.

Sometimes the kidney failure suddenly occurs. In this case, it is called an acute failure of the kidney. An injury, infection, or something else may be the cause. Acute renal failure is often treated with urgency by dialysis for some time. Often, kidney function recovers itself. Generally, this disease settles slowly and silently, but it progresses over the years. People with CKD do not necessarily go from stage 1 to stage 5 of the disease. Stage 5 of the disease is known under the end-stage renal disease (ESRD) or kidney failure in the final stage.

It is important to know that the expressions terminal, final, and ultimate mean the end of any kidneys' function (kidneys working at less than 15% of their normal capacity) and not the end of your life. To stay alive at this stage of the disease, it is necessary to resort to dialysis or a kidney transplant. Dialysis and transplantation are known as renal replacement therapy (TRS).

This means that dialysis or the transplanted kidney will "supplement" or "replace" the sick kidneys and do their job.

Epidemiology - Chronic Kidney Disease: Classification, Risk Factors, and History

Definition and Classification of Chronic Renal Disease

The CKD is defined by the presence of an anatomical and urinary indicator of renal impairment or a decrease in the rate of glomerular filtration (GFR) persisting beyond three months. This disease is classified into five stages of increasing severity, according to the GFR. A DFG within normal limits characterizes the first two stages. It requires renal impairment markers, including urinary tests (proteinuria, Haematuria, or pyuria) or morphological abnormalities renal ultrasound (contours bumpy, asymmetrical in size, small kidneys or large kidneys, polycystic, etc.).

A real decrease in GFR characterizes only the other three stages. The end-stage of chronic renal failure (CRT) or stage 5 of the CKD is defined by a GFR <15 ml/min / 1.73 m².

Renal impairment is defined by the presence of pathological abnormalities or biological markers of the kidney, including abnormalities of urinary or kidney morphological tests detected by imaging.

Historically, the lack of consensus in the definition of CKD (especially chronic renal failure), its severity has led to late diagnosis, inadequate medical management, and data deficiency. Epidemiologically comparable at the global level.

It was not until 2002 that this gap was filled by adopting the DFG thresholds or the CKD mentioned above stages.

What Are the Symptoms of Kidney Disease?

In chronic kidney disease, the deterioration of kidney function is gradual. At the very beginning of the CKD, there are hardly any warning signs or apparent symptoms. In some cases, it is difficult to detect any evidence while the kidneys are already severely affected.

Laboratory analysis of proteins and blood in the urine (urine analysis) can show at an early stage whether the kidney is affected or not. The calculation of serum creatinine levels makes it possible to know, well before other signs occur, whether the kidneys function well or not, or whether there is a decrease in renal function.

Warning signs or symptoms of kidney disease:
- High blood pressure
- The swelling of the eyes, hands, and feet
- Blood in the urine, cloudy or dark urine such as tea
- The presence of proteins in the urine
- Urines foamier than normal
- Less urine or difficulty urinating
- Fatigue, difficulty concentrating
- Loss of appetite or weight
- Generalized and persistent itching

Who Runs the Risk of Having a CKD?

Even though people with diabetes use insulin by injection or take medication, they cannot shelter the lesion of some small blood vessels, like those in the eye's retina. In this case, the retina may be damaged, resulting in loss of vision. Also, they are not immune to the deterioration of the fragile blood vessels of the renal filters.

Progressive deterioration of the kidneys is seen when urine tests show higher and higher protein levels. As the disease progresses, the number of protein increases. As for treatment, the sooner it starts (for example, with drugs such as ACE inhibitors or A2 blocking agents), the more likely it is to slow the disease's progression. Kidney disease caused by diabetes can slow the evolution of the disease regardless of its stage.

Over time, diabetes can reach kidney filters at a point of no return: the kidneys no longer function, and renal replacement therapy becomes essential. People with diabetes are prone to infections, which are changing rapidly. If these infections, especially those of the urinary tract, are not treated, they can damage the kidneys.

Hypertension

The kidneys secrete a hormone that plays an important role in increasing or reducing blood pressure. When the kidneys are so affected that they do not function properly, the secretion of this hormone can increase and cause hypertension, which damages the kidneys. Therefore, it is necessary to closely monitor hypertension to avoid the deterioration of renal function in the long term.

Glomerulonephritis

The glomerulonephritis, or nephritis, occurs when glomeruli, these little tiny filters used to purify the blood, deteriorate. There are several kinds of glomerulonephritis. Some are hereditary, while others occur as a result of certain diseases such as strep throat. The causes of most glomerulonephritis are not yet known. Some glomerulonephritis cure without medical treatment, while others require prescription drugs. Some do not respond to any treatment. Some clues suggest that glomerulonephritis is due to a deficiency in the immune system of the body.

Autosomal Dominant Polycystic Disease
Often in their forties, people with the disease will need dialysis or a kidney transplant. But because the loss of kidney function is changing at a different pace, depending on the individual, the time between the onset of cysts and the need for dialysis varies widely. Since the disease is hereditary, people are advised to inform other family members to carry out the required tests as they may also be affected.

The Obstruction of the Urinary Tract
Any obstruction (or blockage) of the urinary tract may damage the kidneys. Obstructions can occur in the ureter or at the end of the bladder. Narrowing the ureter at the superior or inferior level is sometimes due to congenital malformations, leading to chronic kidney disease in children. In adults, increased prostate volume, kidney stones, or tumors often obstruct the urinary tract.

Reflux Nephropathy
The reflux nephropathy is the new name of the former "chronic pyelonephritis."

Illegal Drugs
The use of illegal drugs can cause kidney damage. Over-the-counter medications (without a prescription) and high-dose and long-term use of over-the-counter medications can cause kidney damage.

Important: Beware of medications, including herbal remedies, sold without a prescription.

Prescription Drugs
Some medications prescribed to people with kidney disease cause renal dysfunction. The lesions are sometimes reversible and sometimes irreversible. Many medications prescribed by prescription are safe but provided the doctor makes changes accurate to the dosage. So always ask your doctor or your pharmacist, information about potential side effects of prescribed drugs.

Other Kidney Disorders
Other issues can affect the kidneys, such as, for example, kidney stones, Syndrome Alport, Fabry disease, Wilms tumor (children only), not including infections of bacterial origin.

CHAPTER 2:

What You Can Eat and What You Should Avoid in Renal Diet

We have established the importance of a renal diet and why you should include it in your lifestyle. Most people assume that it's difficult to follow the renal diet, but it's easier than you think. To get the best results (improved kidney function, reduced dialysis risk), it is important to learn more about kidney disease diet. When you learn what to eat and avoid, it becomes a lot easier to adjust your eating habits. So, before we start cooking some delicious foods, we will go through the list of foods you should eat and avoid managing kidney disease.

It's important to repeat that diet restrictions vary according to the stage of kidney disease. Renal diet usually involves limiting potassium and sodium consumption to 2000 mg a day and lowering phosphorus intake to 1000 mg per day.

Foods to Eat

When it comes to a renal diet, you must opt for low sodium, potassium, phosphorus, and protein.

- Cauliflower – anti-inflammatory properties, abundant in vitamin C, vitamin K, and folate.
- Blueberries – nutrient-rich and abundant in antioxidants that decrease the risk of diabetes, heart disease, and cognitive decline.
- Sea bass – high-quality protein and a good source of Omega-3 fatty acids.
- Red grapes – rich in vitamin C and other valuable nutrients.
- Egg whites – a kidney-friendly source of protein.
- Garlic – a delicious alternative to salt.
- Buckwheat – nutritious, rich in fiber, magnesium, iron, and B vitamins.
- Olive oil – phosphorus-free.
- Bulgur – kidney-friendly alternative to whole grains.
- Cabbage – a source of vitamin K, vitamin C, and B-complex vitamins.
- Skinless chicken – contains less phosphorus, sodium, and potassium than chicken with skin on (remember, an adequate amount of protein is important for your health).
- Bell peppers – low in potassium.
- Onions – sodium-free flavor for renal diet.
- Arugula – nutrient-dense green vegetable low in potassium.
- Macadamia nuts – low in phosphorus.
- Radish – low in potassium and phosphorus.

- Turnip – excellent replacement for high-potassium vegetables such as potatoes.
- Pineapple – low potassium content.
- Cranberries – contain nutrients that prevent bacteria from sticking to the lining of the bladder and urinary tract to cut the risk of infections.
- Shiitake mushrooms – a plant-based meat substitute.
- Apples – high in fiber and anti-inflammatory compounds.

Foods to Avoid

To follow the renal diet that will support kidney function and not disrupt it, you may want to avoid consuming the following foods:

- Avocado – while they are healthy, avocadoes are abundant in potassium.
- Canned foods – contain high amounts of sodium.
- Whole-wheat bread – due to its phosphorus and potassium content.
- Brown rice – high in potassium and phosphorus.
- Bananas – abundant in potassium.
- Dairy – a natural source of phosphorus, potassium, protein.
- Oranges (and OJ) – a rich source of potassium.
- Processed meat – contain high amounts of salt.
- Olives, pickles, and relish – too much salt.
- Apricots – high in potassium.
- Potatoes and sweet potatoes – contain high levels of potassium.
- Tomatoes – high in potassium.
- Instant, packaged, and premade meals – abundant in sodium.
- Spinach, beet greens, Swiss chard – contain high amounts of potassium.
- Prunes, raisins, and dates – abundant in potassium.
- Crackers, chips, pretzels, and other snacks – high in salt.

NOTE: Some foods such as potatoes and sweet potatoes can be leached or soaked to reduce potassium content.

Fluids and Juices for Healthy Kidneys

Management of kidney disease also requires paying attention to fluid intake and the things you drink. For example, you should avoid soda, especially dark-colored cola. But, here are some drinks you should include in your lifestyle:

- Cranberry juice – beneficial for urinary and kidney health.
- Lemon- and lime-based or other citrus juice – kidney stone prevention.
- Water – allows kidneys to filter waste and toxins from the blood.
- Stinging nettle tea – antioxidant-rich, reduces inflammation.

Here and now that you know what to eat and avoid on the renal diet, it's time to start cooking. In the next chapters, you will see some of the best, easiest, and most delicious recipes you can make. The 14-day meal plan is coming right up; scroll down to see more.

CHAPTER 3:

Breakfast

1. Berry Chia with Yogurt
Preparation Time: 35 minutes
Cooking Time: 5 minutes
Servings: 4
Ingredients:
- ½ cup chia seeds, dried
- 2 cup Plain yogurt
- 1/3 cup strawberries, chopped
- ¼ cup blackberries
- ¼ cup raspberries
- 4 teaspoons Splenda

Directions:
1. Mix up together Plain yogurt with Splenda and chia seeds.
2. Transfer the mixture into the serving ramekins (jars) and leave for 35 minutes.
3. After this, add blackberries, raspberries, and strawberries. Mix up the meal well.

Nutrition:
- Calories: 257 Fat: 10.3 g
- Fiber: 11 g
- Carbs: 27.2 g
- Protein: 12 g

2. Arugula Eggs with Chili Peppers
Preparation Time: 7 minutes
Cooking Time: 10 minutes
Servings: 4
Ingredients:
- 2 cups arugula, chopped
- 3 eggs, beaten
- ½ chili pepper, chopped
- 1 tablespoon butter
- 1 oz Parmesan, grated

Directions:
1. Toss butter in the skillet and melt it.
2. Add arugula and sauté it over medium heat for 5 minutes. Stir it from time to time.
3. Meanwhile, mix up together Parmesan, chili pepper, and eggs.
4. Pour the egg mixture over the arugula and scramble well.
5. Cook the breakfast for 5 minutes more over medium heat.

Nutrition:
- Calories: 98
- Fat: 7.8 g
- Fiber: 0.2 g
- Carbs: 0.9 g
- Protein: 6.7 g

3. Breakfast Skillet
Preparation Time: 7 minutes
Cooking Time: 25 minutes
Servings: 5
Ingredients:
- 1 cup cauliflower, chopped
- 1 tablespoon olive oil
- ½ red onion, diced
- 1 tablespoon Plain yogurt

- ½ teaspoon ground black pepper
- 1 teaspoon dried cilantro
- 1 teaspoon dried oregano
- 1 bell pepper, chopped
- 1/3 cup milk
- ½ teaspoon Za'atar
- 1 tablespoon lemon juice
- 1 russet potato, chopped

Directions:
1. Pour olive oil into the skillet and preheat it.
2. Add chopped russet potato and roast it for 5 minutes.
3. After this, add cauliflower, ground black pepper, cilantro, oregano, and bell pepper.
4. Roast the mixture for 10 minutes over medium heat.
5. Then add milk, Za'atar, and Plain Yogurt. Stir it well.
6. Sauté the mixture 10 minutes.
7. Top the cooked meal with diced red onion and sprinkle with lemon juice.
8. It is recommended to serve the breakfast hot.

Nutrition:
- Calories: 112
- Fat: 3.4 g
- Fiber: 2.6 g
- Carbs: 18.1 g
- Protein: 3.1 g

4. Eggplant Chicken Sandwich

Preparation Time: 10 minutes
Cooking Time: 15 minutes
Servings: 2
Ingredients:
- 1 eggplant, trimmed
- 10 oz chicken fillet
- 1 teaspoon Plain yogurt
- ½ teaspoon minced garlic
- 1 tablespoon fresh cilantro, chopped
- 2 lettuce leaves
- 1 teaspoon olive oil
- ½ teaspoon salt
- ½ teaspoon chili pepper
- 1 teaspoon butter

Directions:
1. Slice the eggplant lengthwise into 4 slices.
2. Rub the eggplant slices with minced garlic and brush with olive oil.
3. Grill the eggplant slices on the preheated to 375F grill for 3 minutes from each side.
4. Meanwhile, rub the chicken fillet with salt and chili pepper.
5. Place it in the skillet and add butter.
6. Roast the chicken for 6 minutes from each side over medium-high heat.
7. Cool the cooked eggplants gently and spread one side of them with Plain yogurt.
8. Add lettuce leaves and chopped fresh cilantro.
9. After this, slice the cooked chicken fillet and add over the lettuce.
10. Cover it with the remaining sliced eggplant to get the sandwich shape. Pin the sandwich with the toothpick if needed.

Nutrition:
- Calories: 368
- Fat: 15.2 g
- Fiber: 8.2 g
- Carbs: 14.2 g
- Protein: 43.5 g

5. Panzanella Salad

Preparation Time: 10 minutes
Cooking Time: 5 minutes
Servings: 4
Ingredients:
- 2 cucumbers, chopped
- 1 red onion, sliced
- 2 red bell peppers, chopped
- ¼ cup fresh cilantro, chopped
- 1 tablespoon capers
- 1 oz whole-grain bread, chopped
- 1 tablespoon canola oil
- ½ teaspoon minced garlic
- 1 tablespoon Dijon mustard
- 1 teaspoon olive oil
- 1 teaspoon lime juice

Directions:
1. Pour canola oil into the skillet and bring it to boil.
2. Add chopped bread and roast it until crunchy (3-5 minutes).
3. Meanwhile, in the salad bowl, combine sliced red onion, cucumbers, bell peppers, cilantro, capers, and mix up gently.
4. Make the dressing: mix up together lime juice, olive oil, Dijon mustard, and minced garlic.
5. Transfer the dressing over the salad and stir it directly before serving.

Nutrition:
- Calories: 136
- Fat: 5.7 g
- Fiber: 4.1 g
- Carbs: 20.2 g
- Protein: 4.1 g

6. Shrimp Bruschetta

Preparation Time: 15 minutes
Cooking Time: 10 minutes
Servings: 4
Ingredients:
- 13 oz shrimps, peeled
- 1 tablespoon tomato sauce
- ½ teaspoon Splenda
- ¼ teaspoon garlic powder
- 1 teaspoon fresh parsley, chopped
- ½ teaspoon olive oil
- 1 teaspoon lemon juice
- 4 bread slices
- 1 cup water, for cooking

Directions:
1. Transfer water to the saucepan and bring it to a boil.
2. Add shrimps and boil them over the high heat for 5 minutes.
3. After this, drain shrimps and chill them to room temperature.
4. Mix up together shrimps with Splenda, garlic powder, tomato sauce, and fresh parsley.
5. Add lemon juice and stir gently.
6. Preheat the oven to 360F.
7. Put the bread slices with olive oil and bake for 3 minutes.
8. Then place the shrimp mixture on the bread. The bruschetta is cooked.

Nutrition:
- Calories: 199
- Fat: 3.7 g
- Fiber: 2.1 g
- Carbs: 15.3 g
- Protein: 24.1 g

7. Strawberry Muesli

Preparation Time: 10 minutes
Cooking Time: 30 minutes
Servings: 4
Ingredients:
- 2 cups Greek yogurt
- 1 ½ cup strawberries, sliced
- 1 ½ cup Muesli
- 4 teaspoon maple syrup
- ¾ teaspoon ground cinnamon

Directions:
1. Put Greek yogurt in the food processor.
2. Add 1 cup of strawberries, maple syrup, and ground cinnamon.
3. Blend the ingredients until you get smooth mass.
4. Transfer the yogurt mass to the serving bowls.
5. Add Muesli and stir well.
6. Leave the meal for 30 minutes in the fridge.
7. After this, decorate it with the remaining sliced strawberries.

Nutrition:
- Calories: 149 Fat: 2.6 g
- Fiber: 3.6 g Carbs: 21.6 g
- Protein: 12 g

8. Yogurt Bulgur

Preparation Time: 10 minutes
Cooking Time: 15 minutes
Servings: 3
Ingredients:
- 1 cup bulgur - 2 cups Greek yogurt
- 1 ½ cup water - ½ teaspoon salt
- 1 teaspoon olive oil

Directions:
1. Pour olive oil into the saucepan and add bulgur.
2. Roast it over medium heat for 2-3 minutes. Stir it from time to time.
3. After this, add salt and water.
4. Close the lid and cook bulgur for 15 minutes over medium heat.
5. Then chill the cooked bulgur well and combine it with Greek yogurt. Stir it carefully.
6. Transfer the cooked meal into the serving plates. The yogurt bulgur tastes the best when it is cold.

Nutrition:
- Calories: 274 Fat: 4.9 g
- Fiber: 8.5 g Carbs: 40.8 g
- Protein: 19.2 g

9. Chia Pudding

Preparation Time: 10 minutes
Cooking Time: 30 minutes
Servings: 2
Ingredients:
- ½ cup raspberries
- 2 teaspoons maple syrup
- 1 ½ cup Plain yogurt
- ¼ teaspoon ground cardamom
- 1/3 cup Chia seeds, dried

Directions:
1. Mix up together Plain yogurt with maple syrup and ground cardamom.
2. Add Chia seeds. Stir it gently.
3. Put the yogurt in the serving glasses and top with the raspberries.
4. Refrigerate the breakfast for at least 30 minutes or overnight.

Nutrition:
- Calories: 303 Fat: 11.2 g
- Fiber: 11.8 g Carbs: 33.2 g
- Protein: 15.5 g

10. Yufka Pies

Preparation Time: 15 minutes
Cooking Time: 20 minutes
Servings: 6
Ingredients:
- 7 oz yufka dough/phyllo dough
- 1 cup fresh cilantro, chopped
- 2 eggs, beaten
- 1 teaspoon paprika
- ¼ teaspoon chili flakes
- ½ teaspoon salt
- 2 tablespoons sour cream
- 1 teaspoon olive oil

Directions:
1. In the mixing bowl, combine sour cream, salt, chili flakes, paprika, and beaten eggs.
2. Brush the springform pan with olive oil.
3. Place ¼ part of all yufka dough in the pan and sprinkle it with ¼ part of the egg mixture.
4. Add ¼ cup of cilantro.
5. Cover the mixture with 1/3 part of the remaining yufka dough and repeat all the steps again. You should get 4 layers.
6. Cut the yufka mixture into 6 pies and bake at 360F for 20 minutes. The cooked pies should have a golden brown color.

Nutrition:
- Calories: 213
- Fat: 11.4 g
- Fiber: 0.8 g
- Carbs: 18.2 g
- Protein: 9.1 g

11. Egg White Scramble

Preparation Time: 10 minutes
Cooking Time: 6 hours
Servings: 4
Ingredients:
- 1 teaspoon almond butter
- 4 egg whites
- ¼ teaspoon salt
- ½ teaspoon paprika
- 2 tablespoons heavy cream

Directions:
1. Whisk the egg whites gently and add heavy cream.
2. Put the almond butter in the skillet and melt it.
3. Then add egg white mixture.
4. Sprinkle it with salt and cook for 2 minutes over medium heat.
5. After this, scramble the egg whites with the fork or spatula's help and sprinkle with paprika.
6. Cook the scrambled egg whites for 3 minutes more.
7. Transfer the meal to the serving plates.

Nutrition:
- Calories: 68 Fat: 5.1 g
- Fiber: 0.5 g
- Carbs: 1.3 g
- Protein: 4.6 g

12. Beet Smoothie

Preparation Time: 10 minutes
Cooking Time: 0 minutes
Servings: 2
Ingredients:
- 10 ounces' almond milk, unsweetened
- 2 beets, peeled and quartered
- ½ cup cherries, pitted
- 1 tablespoon almond butter

Directions:
1. In your blender, mix the milk with the beets, cherries, and butter. Pulse well, pour into glasses, and serve.
2. Enjoy!

Nutrition:
- Calories: 165
- Fat: 5 g
- Fiber: 6 g
- Carbs: 22 g
- Protein: 5 g

13. Chia Bars

Preparation Time: 4 hours
Cooking Time: 0 minutes
Servings: 4
Ingredients:
- ½ cup chia seeds
- 1/3 cup cocoa powder
- ½ cup shredded coconut, unsweetened
- 1 cup chopped walnuts
- ½ cup oats
- ½ cup dark chocolate, chopped
- 1 teaspoon vanilla extract

Directions:
1. In your food processor, mix the chia seeds, cocoa, coconut, walnuts, oats, chocolate, and vanilla. Pulse well, then press into a lined baking dish. Keep in the freezer for 4 hours, cut into 12 bars, and serve for breakfast.
2. Enjoy!

Nutrition:
- Calories: 125
- Fat: 5 g
- Fiber: 4 g
- Carbs: 12 g
- Protein: 5 g

14. Pineapple Smoothie

Preparation Time: 10 minutes
Cooking Time: 0 minutes
Servings: 1
Ingredients:
- 1 cup coconut water
- 1 orange, peeled and cut into quarters
- 1½ cups pineapple chunks
- 1 tablespoon fresh grated ginger
- 1 teaspoon chia seeds
- 1 teaspoon turmeric powder
- A pinch of black pepper

Directions:
1. In your blender, mix the coconut water with the orange, pineapple, ginger, chia seeds, turmeric, and black pepper. Pulse well, pour into a glass, and serve for breakfast.

Nutrition:
- Calories: 151
- Fat: 2 g
- Fiber: 6 g
- Carbs: 12 g
- Protein: 4 g

15. Cauliflower Rice and Coconut

Preparation Time: 20 minutes
Cooking Time: 20 minutes
Servings: 4
Ingredients:
- 3 cups of cauliflower, riced
- 2/3 cups of full-fat coconut milk
- 1-2 teaspoons of sriracha paste
- ¼- ½ teaspoon of onion powder
- Salt as needed
- Fresh basil for garnish

Directions:
1. Take a pan and place it over medium-low heat.

2. Add all of the ingredients and stir them until fully combined.
3. Cook for about 5–10 minutes, making sure that the lid is on.
4. Remove the lid and keep cooking until there's no excess liquid.
5. Once the rice is soft and creamy, enjoy it!

Nutrition:
- Calories: 95
- Fat: 7 g
- Carbohydrates: 4 g
- Protein: 1 g

16. Kale and Garlic Platter
Preparation Time: 5 minutes
Cooking Time: 10 minutes
Servings: 4
Ingredients:
- 1 bunch of kale
- 2 tablespoons of oil
- 4 garlic cloves, minced

Directions:
1. Carefully tear the kale into bite-sized portions, making sure to remove the stem.
2. Discard the stems.
3. Take a large-sized pot and put it over medium heat.
4. Add oil and let it heat up.
5. Add garlic and stir for 2 minutes.
6. Add kale and cook for 5–10 minutes.
7. Serve!

Nutrition:
- Calories: 121
- Fat: 8 g
- Carbohydrates: 5 g
- Protein: 4 g

17. Lemon and Broccoli Platter
Preparation Time: 10 minutes
Cooking Time: 15 minutes
Servings: 6
Ingredients:
- 2 heads of broccoli, separated into florets
- 2 teaspoons of extra virgin olive oil
- 1 teaspoon of salt
- ½ teaspoon of black pepper
- 1 garlic clove, minced
- ½ teaspoon of lemon juice

Directions:
1. Preheat your oven to 400°F.
2. Take a large-sized bowl and add broccoli florets.
3. Drizzle olive oil and season with pepper, salt, and garlic.
4. Spread the broccoli out in a single even layer on a baking sheet.
5. Bake for 15–20 minutes until fork tender.
6. Squeeze lemon juice on top.
7. Serve and enjoy!

Nutrition:
- Calories: 49 Fat: 1.9 g
- Carbohydrates: 7 g
- Protein: 3 g

18. Garlic and Butter-Flavored Cod
Preparation Time: 5 minutes
Cooking Time: 20 minutes
Servings: 3
Ingredients:
- 3 Cod fillets, 8 ounces each
- ¾ pound of baby bok choy halved
- 1/3 cup of almond butter, thinly sliced
- 1 ½ tablespoon of garlic, minced
- Salt and pepper to taste

Directions:
1. Preheat your oven to 400°F.
2. Cut 3 sheets of aluminum foil (large enough to fit fillet).
3. Place cod fillet on each sheet and add butter and garlic on top.
4. Add bok choy, season with pepper and salt.
5. Fold packet and enclose them in pouches.
6. Arrange on the baking sheet.
7. Bake for 20 minutes.
8. Let it cool.

Nutrition:
- Calories: 355
- Fat: 21 g
- Carbohydrates: 3 g
- Protein: 37 g

19. Egg White and Pepper Omelet
Preparation Time: 5 minutes
Cooking Time: 5 minutes
Servings: 1–2
Ingredients:
- 4 egg whites, lightly beaten
- 1 red bell pepper, diced
- 1 tsp. of paprika
- 2 tbsp. of olive oil
- ½ tsp. of salt
- Pepper

Directions:
1. In a shallow pan (around 8 inches), heat the olive oil and sauté the bell peppers until softened.
2. Add the egg whites and the paprika, fold the edges into the fluid center with a spatula and let the omelet cook until eggs are fully opaque and solid.
3. Season with salt and pepper.

Nutrition:
- Calories: 165 Carbohydrate: 3.8 g
- Protein: 9.2 g Sodium: 797 mg
- Potassium: 193 mg
- Phosphorus: 202.5 mg
- Dietary Fiber: 0.7 g Fat: 15.22 g

20. Italian Apple Fritters
Preparation Time: 5 minutes
Cooking Time: 8 minutes
Servings: 4
Ingredients:
- 2 large apples, seeded, peeled, and thickly sliced in circles
- 3 tbsp. of corn flour
- ½ tsp. of water
- 1 tsp. of sugar
- 1 tsp. of cinnamon
- Vegetable oil (for frying)
- Sprinkle of icing sugar or honey

Directions:
1. Combine the corn flour, water, and sugar to make your batter in a small bowl.
2. Deep the apple rounds into the corn flour mix.
3. Heat enough vegetable oil to cover half of the pan's surface over medium to high heat.
4. Add the apple rounds into the pan and cook until golden brown.
5. Transfer into a shallow dish with absorbing paper on top and sprinkle with cinnamon and icing sugar.

Nutrition:
- Calories: 183 Carbohydrate: 17.9 g
- Protein: 0.3 g Sodium: 2 g
- Potassium: 100 mg
- Phosphorus: 12.5 mg
- Dietary Fiber: 1.4 g Fat: 14.17 g

21. Tofu and Mushroom Scramble

Preparation Time: 5 minutes
Cooking Time: 4 minutes
Servings: 2
Ingredients:
- ½ cup of sliced white mushrooms
- ⅓ cup of medium-firm tofu, crumbled
- 1 tbsp. of chopped shallots
- ⅓ tsp. of turmeric
- 1 tsp. of cumin
- ⅓ tsp. of smoked paprika
- ½ tsp. of garlic salt
- Pepper
- 3 tbsp. of vegetable oil

Directions:
1. Heat the oil frying pan, set it on a medium, and sauté the sliced mushrooms with the shallots until softened (around 3–4 minutes) over medium to high heat.
2. Add the tofu pieces and toss in the spices and the garlic salt. Toss lightly until tofu and mushrooms are nicely combined.

Nutrition:
- Calories: 220 Carbohydrate: 2.59 g
- Protein: 3.2 g Sodium: 288 mg
- Potassium: 133.5 mg
- Phosphorus: 68.5 mg
- Dietary Fiber: 1.7 g Fat: 23.7 g

22. Egg Fried Rice

Preparation Time: 10 minutes
Cooking Time: 20 minutes
Servings: 6
Ingredients:
- 1 tablespoon of olive oil
- 1 tablespoon of grated peeled fresh ginger
- 1 teaspoon of minced garlic
- 1 cup of chopped carrots
- 1 scallion, white and green parts, chopped
- 2 tablespoons of chopped fresh cilantro
- 4 cups of cooked rice
- 1 tablespoon of low-sodium soy sauce
- 4 eggs, beaten

Directions:
1. Heat the olive oil.
2. Add the ginger and garlic, and sauté until softened, about 3 minutes.
3. Add the carrots, scallion, and cilantro, and sauté until tender, about 5 minutes.
4. Stir in the rice and soy sauce, and sauté until the rice is heated over 5 minutes.
5. Move the rice over to one side of the skillet, and pour the eggs into the space.
6. Scramble the eggs, then mix them into the rice.
7. Serve hot.
8. Low-sodium tip: Soy sauces, even low-sodium versions, are very salty. If you have the time, making your substitution sauce is simple and effective, even if it does not taste quite the same. Many versions of this diet-friendly sauce are online, with ingredients like vinegar, molasses, garlic, and herbs.

Nutrition:
- Calories: 204 Total fat: 6 g
- Saturated fat: 1 g
- Cholesterol: 141 mg
- Sodium: 223 mg
- Carbohydrates: 29 g Fiber: 1 g
- Phosphorus: 120 mg
- Potassium: 147 mg Protein: 8 g

23. Quick Thai Chicken and Vegetable Curry

Preparation Time: 15 minutes
Cooking Time: 20 minutes
Servings: 4
Ingredients:

- 1 ½ cups cauliflower florets
- 1 clove garlic, minced
- 1 cup light coconut milk
- 1 cup low sodium chicken broth
- 1 lb chicken breasts
- 1 medium bell pepper, julienned
- 1 medium onion, halved and sliced
- 1 tbsp fish sauce or low sodium soy sauce
- 1 tbsp fresh ginger, minced
- 1 tbsp lime juice
- 1 tsp light brown sugar
- 1 tsp red curry paste
- 2 tsp canola oil
- Lime wedges

Directions:

1. Heat oil in a skillet. Sauté the onion and bell pepper for four minutes or until soft.
2. Add the ginger, garlic, and curry paste. Mix, then add the chicken. Sauté for two minutes before adding the coconut milk, broth, brown sugar, and fish sauce.
3. Add the cauliflowers and reduce the heat to medium-low. Boil and stir the mixture occasionally until the chicken is cooked through.
4. Serve immediately with lime wedges.

Nutrition:

- Calories: 394
- Carbs: 11 g
- Protein: 29 g
- Fat: 28 g
- Phosphorus: 316 mg
- Potassium: 745 mg
- Sodium: 252 mg

24. Cajun Stuffed Peppers

Preparation Time: 10 minutes
Cooking Time: 45 minutes
Servings: 6
Ingredients:

- 1 cup of chopped roasted red peppers
- 6 fresh bell peppers
- ½ lb. of ground beef
- ½ lb. of ground pork
- ¼ cup of hot water
- 1 medium onion chopped
- 3 cups of cooked white rice
- ½ tsp. of black pepper
- ½ tsp. of lemon pepper
- 1 tbsp. of dried thyme
- 1 tbsp. of minced garlic

Directions:

1. Preheat oven to 350°F.
2. Take a large pot of water to a boil and drop in the bell peppers.
3. Boil the peppers for 5 minutes. Remove and drain.
4. Arrange the peppers by removing the stem and removing the seeds.
5. In a large skillet, cook the ground meat over medium heat until it is browned.
6. Add the hot water, roasted red peppers, onions, garlic, and spices.
7. Cook for 5 minutes.
8. Add rice and stir to combine and cook for 3 minutes. Remove from the heat and stuff the bell peppers. Put the stuffed peppers on a baking sheet and bake uncovered for 30 minutes.

9. Serve with a garnish of roasted red peppers.

Nutrition:
- Calories: 173.5 Protein: 8.8 g
- Sodium: 27.7 mg Phosphorus: 8.0 mg
- Potassium: 166.1 mg

25. Stuffed Zucchini
Preparation Time: 20 minutes
Cooking Time: 45 minutes
Servings: 8
Ingredients:
- 4 large zucchini
- 2 tbsp. of canola oil
- 1 diced onion
- 1 red bell pepper diced
- 1 cup of shredded carrots
- 1 summer squash diced
- 4 matzo broken into pieces
- 1 tsp. of dried oregano
- 2 tsp. of minced garlic
- 1 tsp. of ground pepper
- 1 lb. of ground chicken, cooked

Directions:
1. Preheat oven to 360°F.
2. Slice zucchini in half, lengthwise, and scoop out insides leaving ¼ inch zucchini on skins.
3. Reserve the insides.
4. Place zucchini halves skin-side down on the baking sheet.
5. In a large skillet over medium heat, warm the oil.
6. Add the onion and sauté for 4 minutes.
7. Add the zucchini insides, the rest of the veggies, the matzo, and the spices.
8. Sauté for 2 minutes.
9. Add the chicken and mix well.
10. Remove from heat and stuff the zucchini with the mixture.
11. Bake for 30 minutes.

Nutrition:
- Calories: 157.0 Protein: 9.5 g
- Sodium: 49.0 mg Phosphorus: 4.4 mg
- Potassium: 236.1 mg

26. Savory Collard Chips
Preparation Time: 5 minutes
Cooking Time: 20 minutes
Servings: 4
Ingredients:
- 1 bunch of collard greens
- 1 teaspoon of extra-virgin olive oil
- Juice of ½ lemon
- ½ teaspoon of garlic powder
- ¼ teaspoon of freshly ground black pepper

Directions:
1. Preheat the oven to 350°F. Line a baking sheet with parchment paper.
2. Cut the collards into 2-by-2-inch squares and pat dry with paper towels.
3. Toss greens with the olive oil, lemon juice, garlic powder, and pepper in a large bowl. Use your hands to combine well, massaging the dressing into the greens until evenly coated.
4. Arrange the collards in a single layer on the baking sheet, and cook for 8 minutes.

Nutrition:
- Calories: 24 Total Fat: 1 g
- Saturated Fat: 0 g
- Cholesterol: 0 mg
- Carbohydrates: 3 g Fiber: 1 g
- Protein: 1 g Phosphorus: 6 mg
- Potassium: 72 mg Sodium: 8 mg

27. Blackberry Pudding
Preparation Time: 45 minutes
Cooking Time: 30 minutes
Servings: 2
Ingredients:
- ¼ cup chia seeds
- ½ cup blackberries, fresh
- 1 teaspoon liquid sweetener
- 1 cup coconut milk, full fat and unsweetened
- 1 teaspoon vanilla extract

Directions:
1. Take the vanilla, liquid sweetener, and coconut milk and add to the blender.
2. Process until thick.
3. Add blackberries and process until smooth.
4. Divide the mixture between cups and chill for 30 minutes.
5. Serve and enjoy!

Nutrition:
- Calories: 437
- Fat: 38 g
- Carbohydrates: 8 g
- Protein: 8

28. Simple Green Shake
Preparation Time: 5 minutes
Cooking Time: 10 minutes
Servings: 1
Ingredients:
- ¾ cup whole milk yogurt
- 2½ cups lettuce, mix salad greens
- 1 pack stevia
- 1 tablespoon MCT oil
- 1 tablespoon chia seeds
- 1 ½ cups of water

Directions:
1. Add listed ingredients to a blender.
2. Combine until you have a creamy texture.
3. Serve chilled and enjoy!

Nutrition:
- Calories: 320
- Fat: 24 g
- Carbohydrates: 17 g
- Protein: 10 g

29. Fine Morning Porridge
Preparation Time: 15 minutes
Cooking Time: 10 minutes
Servings: 2
Ingredients:
- 2 tablespoons coconut flour
- 2 tablespoons vanilla protein powder
- 3 tablespoons Golden Flaxseed meal
- 1 ½ cups almond milk, unsweetened
- Powdered erythritol

Directions:
1. Take a bowl and mix in flaxseed meal, protein powder, coconut flour, and mix well.
2. Add mix to the saucepan (placed over medium heat).
3. Add almond milk and stir; let the mixture thicken.
4. Add your desired amount of sweetener and serve.

Nutrition:
- Calories: 259
- Fat: 13 g
- Carbohydrates: 5 g
- Protein: 16 g

30. Hungarian's Porridge

Preparation Time: 10 minutes
Cooking Time: 10 minutes
Servings: 2
Ingredients:
- 1 tablespoon chia seeds
- 1 tablespoon ground flaxseed
- 1/3 cup coconut cream
- ½ cup of water
- 1 teaspoon vanilla extract
- 1 tablespoon almond butter

Directions:
1. Add chia seeds, coconut cream, flaxseed, water, and vanilla to a small pot.
2. Mix and let it sit for 6 minutes.
3. Put butter and place pot over low heat.
4. Keep stirring as butter melts.
5. Once the porridge is hot/not boiling, pour into a bowl.
6. Add a few berries or a dash of cream for extra flavor.

Nutrition:
- Calories: 410
- Fat: 38 g
- Carbohydrates: 10 g
- Protein: 6 g

31. Zucchini and Onion Platter

Preparation Time: 15 minutes
Cooking Time: 45 minutes
Servings: 4
Ingredients:
- 3 large zucchinis, julienned
- ½ cup basil
- 2 red onions, thinly sliced
- ¼ teaspoon salt
- 1 teaspoon cayenne pepper
- 2 tablespoons lemon juice

Directions:
1. Create zucchini Zoodles by using a vegetable peeler and shaving the zucchini with the peeler lengthwise until you get to the core and seeds.
2. Turn zucchini and repeat until you have long strips.
3. Discard seeds.
4. Lay strips on the cutting board and slice lengthwise to your desired thickness.
5. Mix Zoodles in a bowl alongside onion, basil, and toss.
6. Sprinkle salt and cayenne pepper on top.
7. Drizzle lemon juice.

Nutrition:
- Calories: 156
- Fat: 8 g
- Carbohydrates: 6 g
- Protein: 7 g

32. Collard Greens Dish

Preparation Time: 10 minutes
Cooking Time: 60 minutes
Servings: 6
Ingredients:
- 1 tablespoon olive oil
- 3 slices of bacon, sliced
- 1 large onion, chopped
- 2 garlic cloves, minced
- 1 teaspoon salt
- 3 cups chicken broth
- 1 red pepper flake
- 1-pound fresh collard greens, cut into 2-inch pieces

Directions:
1. Take a large-sized pan.
2. Put oil and allow the oil to heat it up.

3. Add bacon and cook it until crispy and remove it, crumble the bacon and add the crumbled bacon to the pan.
4. Add onion and keep cooking for 5 minutes.
5. Add garlic and cook until you have a nice fragrance.
6. Add collard greens and keep frying until wilted; add chicken broth and season with pepper, salt, and red pepper flakes.
7. Reduce the heat and cover with a lid. Simmer for 45 minutes.
8. Enjoy!

Nutrition:
- Calories: 127
- Fat: 10 g
- Carbohydrates: 8 g
- Protein: 4 g

33. Simple Zucchini BBQ

Preparation Time: 10 minutes
Cooking Time: 10 minutes
Servings: 2
Ingredients:
- Olive oil as needed
- 3 zucchini
- ½ teaspoon black pepper
- ½ teaspoon mustard
- ½ teaspoon cumin
- 1 teaspoon paprika
- 1 teaspoon garlic powder
- 1 tablespoon of sea salt
- 1-2 stevia
- 1 tablespoon chili powder

Directions:
1. Preheat your oven to 300°F.
2. Take a small bowl and add cayenne, black pepper, salt, garlic, mustard, paprika, chili powder, and stevia.
3. Mix well.
4. Slice zucchini into 1/8 inch slices and spray them with olive oil.
5. Sprinkle spice blend over zucchini and bake for 40 minutes.
6. Remove and flip; spray with more olive oil and leftover spice.
7. Bake for 20 minutes more.
8. Serve!

Nutrition:
- Calories: 163
- Fat: 14 g
- Carbohydrates: 3 g
- Protein: 8 g

34. Angel Eggs

Preparation Time: 15 minutes
Cooking Time: 10 minutes
Servings: 2
Ingredients:
- 4 eggs, hardboiled and peeled
- 1 tablespoon vanilla bean sweetener, sugar-free
- 2 tablespoons Keto-Friendly mayonnaise
- 1/8 teaspoon cinnamon

Directions:
1. Halve the boiled eggs and scoop out the yolk.
2. Place in a bowl.
3. Put egg whites on a plate.
4. Add sweetener, cinnamon, and mayo to the egg yolks and mash them well.
5. Transfer the yolk mix to white halves.

Nutrition:
- Calories: 184
- Fat: 15 g
- Carbohydrates: 1 g
- Protein: 12 g

35. Denver Omelets

Preparation Time: 4 minutes
Cooking Time: 1 minute
Servings: 2
Ingredients:
- 2 tablespoons almond butter
- ¼ cup onion, chopped
- ¼ cup green bell pepper, diced
- 2 whole eggs
- ¼ cup ham, chopped

Directions:
1. Put a skillet and place it over medium heat.
2. Add butter and wait until the butter melts.
3. Add onion and bell pepper and sauté for a few minutes.
4. Take a bowl and whip eggs.
5. Add the remaining ingredients and stir.
6. Add sautéed onion and pepper, stir.
7. Microwave the egg mix for 1 minute.

Nutrition:
- Calories: 605
- Fat: 46 g
- Carbohydrates: 6 g
- Protein: 39 g

36. Scrambled Eggs and Pesto

Preparation Time: 5 minutes
Cooking Time: 5 minutes
Servings: 2
Ingredients:
- 3 large whole eggs
- 1 tablespoon almond butter
- 1 tablespoon pesto
- 2 tablespoons creamed coconut milk
- Salt and pepper as needed

Directions:
1. Take a bowl and crack open your egg.
2. Flavor with salt and pepper.
3. Pour eggs into a pan.
4. Add butter and introduce heat.
5. Cook on low heat and gently add pesto.
6. Once the egg is cooked and scrambled, remove it from the heat.
7. Spoon in coconut cream and mix well.
8. Turn on the heat and cook on LOW until you have a creamy texture.
9. Serve and enjoy!

Nutrition:
- Calories: 467
- Fat: 41 g
- Carbohydrates: 3 g
- Protein: 20 g

37. Lemon Broccoli

Preparation Time: 10 minutes
Cooking Time: 15 minutes
Servings: 4
Ingredients:
- 2 heads broccoli, separated into florets
- 2 teaspoons extra virgin olive oil
- 1 teaspoon salt
- ½ teaspoon pepper
- 1 garlic clove, minced
- ½ teaspoon lemon juice

Directions:
1. Preheat your oven to a temperature of 400 °F.
2. Take a large-sized bowl and add broccoli florets with some extra virgin olive oil, pepper, sea salt and garlic.
3. Spread the broccoli out in a single even layer on a fine baking sheet.
4. Bake in your preheated oven for about 15-20 minutes until the florets are soft enough so that they can be pierced with a fork.

5. Squeeze lemon juice over them generously before serving.
6. Enjoy!

Nutrition:
- Calories: 49
- Fat: 2 g
- Carbohydrates: 4 g
- Protein: 3 g

38. Eggplant Fries

Preparation Time: 15 minutes
Cooking Time: 10 minutes
Servings: 8
Ingredients:
- 2 eggs
- 2 cups almond flour
- 2 tablespoons coconut oil, spray
- 2 eggplants, peeled and cut thinly
- Salt and pepper

Directions:
1. Preheat your oven to 400 °F.
2. Take a bowl and mix with salt and black pepper in it.
3. Take another bowl and beat eggs until frothy.
4. Dip the eggplant pieces into the eggs.
5. Then coat them with the flour mixture.
6. Add another layer of flour and egg.
7. Then, take a baking sheet and grease with coconut oil on top.
8. Bake for about 15 minutes.

Nutrition:
- Calories: 212
- Fat: 15.8 g
- Carbohydrates: 12.1 g
- Protein: 8.6 g

39. Pineapple Oatmeal

Preparation Time: 10 minutes
Cooking Time: 4-8 hours
Servings: 5
Ingredients:
- 1 cup steel-cut oats
- 4 cups unsweetened almond milk
- 2 medium apples, slashed
- 1 teaspoon coconut oil
- 1 teaspoon cinnamon
- ¼ teaspoon nutmeg
- 2 tablespoons maple syrup, unsweetened
- A drizzle of lemon juice

Directions:
1. Add the listed ingredients to a cooking pan and mix well.
2. Cook on a very low flame for 8 hours or on high flame for 4 hours.
3. Gently stir
4. Add your desired toppings.
5. Stock in the fridge for later use. Make sure to add a splash of almond milk after re-heating for added flavor.

Nutrition:
- Calories: 180 Fat: 5 g
- Carbohydrates: 31 g
- Protein: 5 g

40. Simple Chia Porridge

Preparation Time: 10 minutes
Cooking Time: 5-10 minutes
Servings: 2
Ingredients:
- 1 tablespoon chia seeds
- 1 tablespoon ground flaxseed
- 1/3 cup coconut cream
- ½ cup of water
- 1 teaspoon vanilla extract
- 1 tablespoon almond butter

Directions:
1. Add chia seeds, coconut cream, flaxseed, water, and vanilla to a small pot.
2. Mix and let it sit for 7 minutes.
3. Put almond butter and place pot over low heat.
4. Keep stirring as almond butter melts.
5. Once the porridge is hot/not boiling, pour into a bowl.
6. Add a few berries or a dash of cream for extra flavor.

Nutrition:
- Calories: 410 Fat: 38 g
- Carbohydrates: 10 g Protein: 6 g

41. Pepperoni Omelet
Preparation Time: 5 minutes
Cooking Time: 20 minutes
Servings: 2
Ingredients:
- 3 eggs
- 7 pepperoni slices
- 1 teaspoon coconut cream
- Salt and ground black pepper, to taste
- 2 tablespoons almond butter

Directions:
1. Take a bowl and whisk eggs with all the remaining ingredients.
2. Then take a skillet and heat the butter.
3. Pour one quarter of the egg mixture into your skillet.
4. After that, cook for 2 minutes per side.
5. Repeat to use the entire batter.

Nutrition:
- Calories: 141
- Fat: 11.5 g
- Carbohydrates: 0.6 g
- Protein: 8.9 g

42. Scrambled Turkey Eggs
Preparation Time: 15 minutes
Cooking Time: 15 minutes
Servings: 2
Ingredients:
- 1 tablespoon coconut oil
- 1 medium red bell pepper, diced
- ½ medium yellow onion, diced
- ¼ teaspoon hot pepper sauce
- 3 large free-range eggs
- ¼ teaspoon black pepper, freshly ground
- ¼ teaspoon salt

Directions:
1. Put a pan to medium-high heat and add coconut oil. Let it heat up
2. Add onions and Sauté
3. Add turkey and red pepper
4. Cook until turkey is cooked
5. Take a bowl and beat eggs, stir in salt and pepper
6. Pour eggs in the pan with turkey and gently cook and scramble eggs
7. Top with hot sauce, and enjoy!

Nutrition:
- Calories: 435
- Fat: 30 g
- Carbohydrates: 34 g
- Protein: 16 g

43. Cinnamon Flavored Baked Apple Chips
Preparation Time: 5 minutes
Cooking Time: 2 hours
Servings: 2
Ingredients:
- 1 teaspoon cinnamon
- 1-2 apples

Directions:
1. Preheat your oven to 200 °F.

2. Take a sharp knife and slice apples into thin slices.
3. Discard seeds.
4. Make sure they do not overlap.
5. Once done, sprinkle cinnamon over the apples.
6. Bake in the oven for 1 hour.
7. Flip and bake for an hour more until no longer moist.

Nutrition:
- Calories: 147
- Fat: 0 g
- Carbohydrates: 39 g
- Protein: 1 g

44. Apple & Cinnamon French Toast

Preparation Time: 20 minutes
Cooking Time: 50 minutes
Servings: 12
Ingredients:
- Cooking spray
- 1 lb. loaf cinnamon raisin bread, cubed
- 1 apple, diced
- 6 tablespoons butter
- 1 teaspoon ground cinnamon
- 8 eggs
- 1 cup half and half
- ¼ cup pancake syrup
- 1 cup almond milk

Directions:
1. Spray oil on a baking dish.
2. Arrange half of the bread cubes.
3. Top with the apples.
4. Sprinkle the cinnamon over the apple and bread.
5. Top with the remaining bread cubes.
6. In a bowl, beat eggs with half and half.
7. Add syrup, almond milk, and butter.
8. Pour mixture over the bread.
9. Cover with foil.
10. Refrigerate for 2 hours.
11. Let cool for 10 minutes before serving.
12. Slice into 12 servings.

Nutrition:
- Calories: 324
- Protein: 9 g
- Carbohydrates: 27 g
- Fat: 20 g
- Cholesterol: 170 mg
- Sodium: 280 mg
- Potassium: 224 mg
- Phosphorus: 150 mg
- Fiber: 1.8 g

45. Blueberry Smoothie in a Bowl

Preparation Time: 15 minutes
Cooking Time: 0 minutes
Servings: 1
Ingredients:
- 1 cup frozen blueberries
- ¼ cup plain Greek yogurt
- 2 tablespoons whey protein powder
- ¼ cup vanilla almond milk (unsweetened)
- 1 tablespoon cereal
- 5 raspberries, sliced
- 2 strawberries, sliced
- 2 teaspoons coconut flakes

Directions:
1. Put the blueberries, yogurt, whey protein powder, and almond milk in a blender.
2. Blend until smooth.
3. Pour mixture into a bowl.
4. Top with cereal, raspberries, and strawberries.

5. Sprinkle coconut flakes on top.

Nutrition:
- Calories: 225
- Protein: 17 g
- Carbohydrates: 28 g
- Fat: 5 g
- Cholesterol: 3 mg
- Sodium: 118 mg
- Potassium 370 mg
- Phosphorus 174 mg
- Calcium 240 mg
- Fiber 7.8 g

46. Egg Pockets

Preparation Time: 15 minutes
Cooking Time: 20 minutes
Servings: 4

Ingredients:
- 1 teaspoon dry yeast
- 1 cup warm water
- 1 tablespoon oil
- 1 teaspoon garlic powder
- 2 cups all-purpose flour
- 1 tablespoon sugar
- 3 eggs, beat
- Cooking spray

Directions:
1. Dissolve the yeast in water.
2. Add the oil, garlic powder, flour, and sugar.
3. Form soft dough from the mixture.
4. Let it sit for 5 minutes.
5. Roll out the dough and slice into 4 portions.
6. Create a bowl with the dough.
7. Beat the eggs.
8. Put the egg on top of the dough.
9. Fold the dough and pinch the edges.
10. Bake in the oven at 350 degrees F for 20 minutes.

Nutrition:
- Calories: 321 Protein: 11 g
- Carbohydrates: 25 g
- Fat: 7 g
- Cholesterol: 123 mg
- Sodium: 50 mg
- Potassium: 139 mg
- Phosphorus: 130 mg
- Calcium: 30 mg Fiber: 2 g

47. Italian Eggs with Peppers

Preparation Time: 15 minutes
Cooking Time: 20 minutes
Servings: 6

Ingredients:
- ½ cup onion, minced
- 1 cup red bell pepper, chopped
- 8 eggs, beaten
- Black pepper to taste
- ¼ cup fresh basil, chopped

Directions:
1. In a skillet, cook onion and red bell pepper until soft.
2. Season eggs with black pepper.
3. Pour egg mixture into the pan.
4. Cook without mixing until firm.
5. Sprinkle fresh basil on top before serving.

Nutrition:
- Calories: 194
- Protein: 13 g
- Carbohydrates: 5 g
- Fat: 14 g
- Cholesterol: 423 mg
- Sodium: 141 mg
- Potassium: 222 mg
- Phosphorus: 203 mg
- Calcium: 64 mg
- Fiber: 0.8 g

48. Mushroom Omelet

Preparation Time: 10 minutes
Cooking Time: 5 minutes
Servings: 2
Ingredients:
- 2 teaspoons butter
- 2 tablespoons onion, chopped
- ½ cup mushroom, diced
- ¼ cup sweet red peppers, chopped
- 3 eggs, beaten
- 1 teaspoon Worcestershire sauce
- ¼ teaspoon black pepper

Directions:
1. Melt butter in a pan over medium heat.
2. Cook the onion, mushroom, and sweet peppers for 5 minutes.
3. Remove from the pan and set aside.
4. Mix the eggs and Worcestershire sauce.
5. Cook eggs over medium heat.
6. When the edges start to become firm, add onion mixture on top.
7. Season with pepper.
8. Fold the omelet.

Nutrition:
- Calories 199
- Protein 11 g
- Carbohydrates 4 g
- Fat 15 g
- Cholesterol 341 mg
- Sodium 276 mg
- Potassium 228 mg
- Phosphorus 167 mg
- Calcium 55 mg
- Fiber 0.6 g

49. Asparagus Frittata

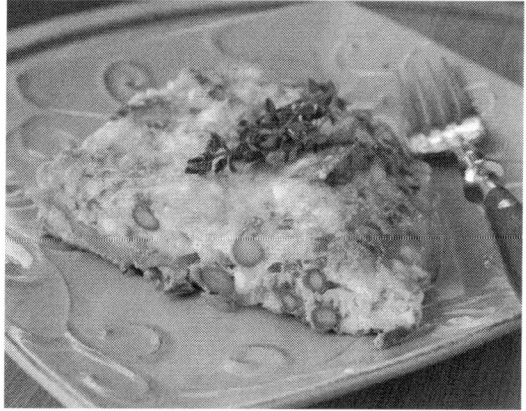

Preparation Time: 5 minutes
Cooking Time: 30 minutes
Servings: 2
Ingredients:
- 10 medium asparagus spears, ends trimmed
- 2 teaspoons extra-virgin olive oil, divided
- Freshly ground black pepper
- 4 large eggs
- ½ teaspoon onion powder
- ¼ cup chopped parsley

Directions:
1. Heat the oven to 350°F.
2. Mix the asparagus with 1 teaspoon of olive oil and season with pepper. Place it in a baking pan and roast, occasionally stirring for 20 minutes until the spears are browned and tender.
3. In a small bowl, beat the eggs with the onion powder and parsley. Season with pepper.
4. Cut the asparagus spears into 1-inch pieces and arrange in a medium skillet. Drizzle with the remaining oil, and shake the pan to distribute.
5. Pour the egg mixture into the skillet, and cook over medium heat. When

the egg is well set on the bottom and nearly set on the top, cover it with a plate, invert the pan, so the frittata is on the plate, and then slide it back into the pan with the cooked side up. Continue to cook for about 30 more seconds, until firm.

Nutrition:
- Calories: 102
- Total Fat: 8 g
- Saturated Fat: 2 g
- Cholesterol: 104 mg
- Carbohydrates: 4 g
- Fiber: 2 g
- Protein: 6 g
- Phosphorus: 103 mg
- Potassium: 248 mg
- Sodium: 46 mg

50. Poached Eggs with Cilantro Butter

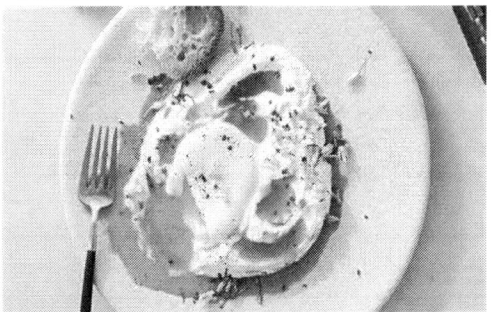

Preparation Time: 5 minutes
Cooking Time: 10 minutes
Servings: 2
Ingredients:
- 2 tablespoons unsalted butter
- 1 tablespoon chopped parsley
- 1 tablespoon chopped cilantro
- 4 large eggs
- Dash vinegar
- Freshly ground black pepper

Directions:
1. In a small pan over low heat, melt the butter. Add the parsley and cilantro, and cook for about 1 minute, stirring constantly. Remove from the heat, and pour into a small dish.
2. In a small saucepan, bring about 3 inches of water to a simmer. Add the dash of vinegar.
3. Crack 1 egg into a cup or ramekin. Using a spoon, create a whirlpool in the simmering water, and then pour the egg into the water. Use the spoon to draw the white together until just starting to set. Repeat with the remaining eggs. Cook for 4 to 7 minutes, depending on how cooked you like your yolk.
4. With a slotted spoon, remove the eggs.
5. Serve the eggs topped with 1 tablespoon of the herbed butter and some pepper.

Nutrition:
- Calories: 261
- Total Fat: 22 g
- Saturated Fat: 7 g
- Cholesterol: 429 mg
- Carbohydrates: 1
- Fiber: 0 g
- Protein: 14 g
- Phosphorus: 226 mg
- Potassium: 173 mg
- Sodium: 164 mg

51. Chorizo and Egg Tortilla

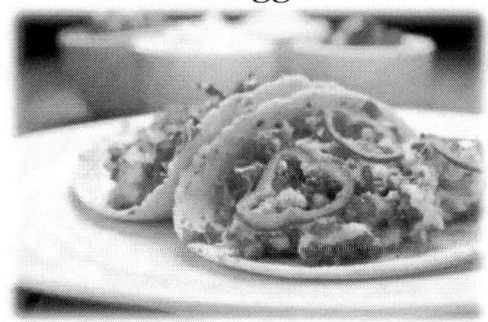

Preparation Time: 10 minutes
Cooking Time: 13 minutes
Servings: 1 tortilla
Ingredients:

- 1 flour tortilla, about 6-inches
- 1/3 cup chorizo meat, chopped
- 1 egg

Directions:

1. Take a medium-sized skillet pan, place it over medium heat, and when hot, add chorizo.
2. When the meat has cooked, drain the excess fat, whisk an egg, pour it into the pan, stir until combined, and cook for 3 minutes, or until eggs have cooked.
3. Spoon egg onto the tortilla and then serve.

Nutrition:

- Calories: 223
- Cholesterol: 211 ml
- Fat: 11 g
- Net Carbs: 13.5 g
- Protein: 16 g
- Sodium: 317 mg
- Carbohydrates: 15 g
- Phosphorus: 232 mg
- Fiber: 1.5 g

52. Cottage Pancakes

Preparation Time: 10 minutes
Cooking Time: 50 minutes
Servings: 6 pancakes
Ingredients:

- 3 cups fresh raspberries, sliced
- ½ cup all-purpose white flour
- 6 tablespoons unsalted butter, melted
- 4 eggs, beaten

Directions:

1. Crack eggs in a medium-sized bowl, add flour, and butter to it, and whisk until combined.
2. Take a medium-high frying pan, grease it with oil and when hot, pour in prepared batter, ¼ cup of batter per pancake, spread the batter into a 4-inch pancake, and cook for 3 minutes per side until browned.
3. When done, transfer pancakes onto a plate, cook more pancakes in the same manner, and, when done, serve each pancake with ½ sliced raspberries.

Nutrition:

- Calories: 253
- Cholesterol: 182 ml
- Fat: 17 g
- Net Carbs: 19 g
- Protein: 11 g
- Sodium: 172 mg
- Carbohydrates: 21 g
- Phosphorus: 159 mg
- Fiber: 2 g

53. Egg in a Hole

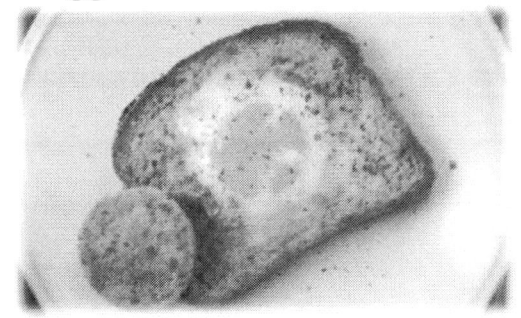

Preparation Time: 5 minutes
Cooking Time: 5 minutes
Servings: 1 slice
Ingredients:

- 1 slice of white bread
- ¼ teaspoon lemon pepper seasoning, salt-free
- 1 egg

Directions:
1. Prepare the bread by making a hole in the middle. Use a cookie cutter for cutting out the center.
2. Brush the slice with oil on both sides, then take a medium-sized skillet pan, place it over medium heat and when hot, add bread slice in it.
3. Crack the egg in the center of the slice sprinkle with lemon pepper seasoning.
4. Cook the egg for 2 minutes, then carefully flip it along with the slice and continue cooking for an additional 2 minutes.

Nutrition:
- Calories: 159 Cholesterol: 213 ml
- Fat: 7 g Net Carbs: 14.2 g
- Protein: 9 g
- Sodium: 266 mg
- Carbohydrates: 15 g
- Phosphorus: 137 mg
- Fiber: 0.8 g

54. German Pancakes

Preparation Time: 10 minutes
Cooking Time: 15 minutes
Servings: 10 pancakes
Ingredients:

- 2/3 cup all-purpose flour
- ¼ teaspoon vanilla extract, unsweetened
- 2 tablespoons white sugar
- 1 cup milk, low-fat
- 4 eggs
- 1/3 cup fruit jam for serving, sugar-free

Directions:
1. Prepare the batter by taking a medium-sized bowl, add flour in it along with sugar, stir until mixed, whisk in eggs until blended, and then whisk in vanilla and milk until smooth.
2. Take a skillet pan, about 8 inches, spray it with oil and when hot, add 3 tablespoons of the prepared batter, tilt the pan to spread the batter evenly
3. Flip the pancake, continue cooking for 45 seconds until the other side is browned, and when done, transfer the pancake to a plate.
4. Cook nine more pancakes in the same manner and, when done on one side of the pancake, fold it and then serve with 1 tablespoon of fruit jam.

Nutrition:
- Calories: 74 Cholesterol: 76 ml
- Fat: 2 g Net Carbs: 0.8 g
- Protein: 4 g
- Sodium: 39 mg
- Carbohydrates: 10 g
- Phosphorus: 76 mg
- Fiber: 0.2 g

55. Mushroom and Red Pepper Omelet

Preparation Time: 5 minutes
Cooking Time: 12 minutes
Servings: 2 plates
Ingredients:

- 2 tablespoons white onion, diced
- ¼ cup sweet red peppers, diced
- ½ cup mushrooms, diced
- ¼ teaspoon ground black pepper
- 1 teaspoon Worcestershire sauce
- 2 teaspoons unsalted butter
- 3 eggs

Directions:
1. Take a medium-sized skillet pan, place it over medium heat, and add 1 teaspoon butter until onions are tender.
2. Stir in red pepper, then transfer vegetables to a plate and set aside until needed.
3. Crack the eggs in a bowl, add Worcestershire sauce, and whisk until combined.
4. Return skillet pan over medium heat, add remaining butter, and when it melts, pour in the egg mixture, and cook for 2 minutes, or until omelet is partially cooked.
5. Then top cooked vegetables on one side of the omelet, and continue cooking until the omelet is cooked completely.
6. When done, remove the pan from the heat, cover the omelet's filling by folding the other half of the omelet, sprinkle it with black pepper, and then divide the omelet into two.
7. Serve straight away.

Nutrition:
- Calories: 199
- Cholesterol: 341 ml
- Fat: 15 g
- Net Carbs: 3.4 g
- Protein: 11 g
- Sodium: 276 mg
- Carbohydrates: 4 g
- Potassium: 228 mg
- Fiber: 0.6 g
- Phosphorus: 167 mg

56. Apple and Zucchini Bread

Preparation Time: 15 minutes
Cooking Time: 50 minutes
Servings: 36 slices
Ingredients:
Loaves:

- 2 cups zucchini, grated
- 3 ½ cups and 2 tablespoons all-purpose white flour
- 1 cup apples, chopped
- 1 ½ teaspoons baking soda
- ¾ cup white sugar
- ½ teaspoon salt
- 3 teaspoons ground cinnamon
- ¾ cup Splenda brown sugar blend
- 1 teaspoon vanilla extract, unsweetened
- ½ cup olive oil
- 4 eggs

Topping:

- ¼ cup all-purpose white flour
- 2 tablespoons unsalted butter, cold
- ¼ cup brown sugar

Directions:
1. Switch on the oven, then set it to 350°F and let it preheat.
2. Meanwhile, take two 9-by-5 inches' loaf pans, spray them with oil, sprinkle

with 2 tablespoons of flour, and set aside until needed.
3. Crack eggs in a large bowl, add vanilla, eggs, oil, white sugar, and ¾ cup brown sugar, and whisk until combined.
4. Take another large bowl, add remaining flour in it, stir in baking soda, 2 tablespoons cinnamon, and salt until mixed. Then, gradually stir the flour mixture into the egg mixture until incorporated. Don't over-mix.
5. Then fold in grated zucchini and chopped apples until mixed, distribute the batter evenly between the two prepared loaf pans and bake in the heated oven for 40 minutes.
6. Meanwhile, prepare the topping by placing all of its ingredients in a food processor and pulse until the mixture resembles crumbs.
7. After 40 minutes of baking, top the loaves evenly with the topping and continue baking for 10 minutes, or until the top has turned golden-brown, and loaves passed the skewer test (if the skewer comes out clean from the center of the bread).
8. When done, let the loaves cool in the pan for 10 minutes, then take them out from the pan and cool them for 20 minutes on the wire rack.
9. Cut each loaf into eighteen slices, each about ½-inch thick, and then serve.

Nutrition:
- Calories: 134 Cholesterol: 25 ml
- Fat: 5 g Net Carbs: 1.4 g
- Protein: 2 g Sodium: 93 mg
- Carbohydrates: 20 g
- Potassium: 53 mg
- Fiber: 0.6 g Phosphorus: 28 mg

57. Spicy Corn Bread
Preparation Time: 15 minutes
Cooking Time: 30 minutes
Servings: 8 pieces
Ingredients:
- ½ cup scallions, chopped
- ¼ teaspoon minced garlic
- ¼ cup carrots, grated
- 1 cup cornmeal
- 1 cup all-purpose white flour
- 2 teaspoons baking powder
- ¼ teaspoon ground black pepper
- 1 tablespoon white sugar
- 1 teaspoon red chili powder
- 1 egg
- 2 tablespoons canola oil
- 1 egg white
- 1 cup of rice milk

Directions:
1. Switch on the oven, then set it to 400°F and let it preheat.
2. Meanwhile, take a large bowl, add cornmeal and flour to it, and then stir in black pepper, red chili powder, baking powder, and sugar until combined.
3. Take another large bowl, add egg and egg white to it, whisk in oil and milk until blended, and then gradually whisk this mixture into the flour mixture until incorporated.
4. Add carrots, scallions, and garlic, stir until just mixed, then take an 8-inch baking pan, grease it with oil, pour the prepared batter in it, and bake for 30 minutes until bread is firm and the top has turned golden-brown.

5. When done, let the bread cool for 10 minutes in the pan, then take it out, cut the bread into eight pieces, each about 2-by-4 inches, and serve.

Nutrition:
- Calories: 188 Cholesterol: 26 ml
- Fat: 5 g Net Carbs: 29 g
- Protein: 5 g Sodium: 155 mg
- Carbohydrates: 31 g
- Potassium: 100 mg
- Fiber: 2 g
- Phosphorus: 81 mg

58. Breakfast Casserole

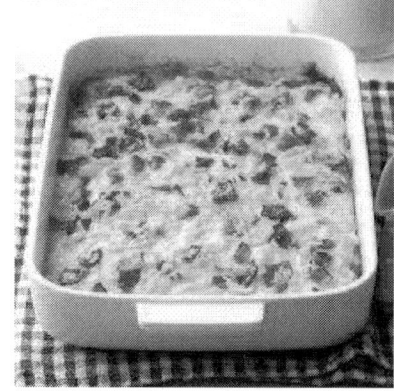

Preparation Time: 10 minutes
Cooking Time: 60 Minutes
Servings: 8
Ingredients:
- 200 grams of lean ground beef – fresh and grass-fed if possible
- 4 slices of bread – white, cut into cubes
- 5 eggs
- 1 teaspoon of mustard – dry
- ½ teaspoon garlic powder with no added sodium

Directions:
1. Preheat your oven to 350 degrees F as you are preparing ingredients for your breakfast casserole.
2. Cube bread slices and place them aside while you are taking care of the ground beef. As you prepare the beef, add a tablespoon of olive oil to the skillet and add the beef.
3. Cook the beef with occasional stirring as you are breaking the meat parts to bits. Once the meat is browned, set aside and add garlic powder, stirring it well to combine.
4. Beat the five eggs in a bowl, combine all ingredients in the egg bowl, and mix to get a homogenous mass out of the egg mixture. Pour the mixture into the mildly greased baking dish and place it in the oven. Bake for 50 minutes or until ready.

Nutrition:
- Potassium: 176 mg
- Sodium: 201 mg
- Phosphorus: 119 mg
- Calories: 220

59. Cauliflower Tortilla

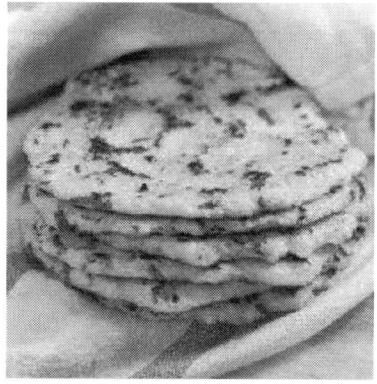

Preparation Time: 15 minutes
Cooking Time: 25 Minutes
Servings: 4
Ingredients:
- 4 cups cauliflower
- 1 cup onion – chopped

- 2 garlic cloves – minced
- 1 cup egg substitute - liquefied
- ¼ teaspoon nutmeg
- 1 tablespoon parsley – fresh, chopped
- ½ teaspoon allspice

Directions:
1. Prepare the cauliflower by cutting it into small cubes, then place the cauliflower bits in a bowl with a tablespoon of water and microwave it for 5 minutes until cauliflower is crisped.
2. While you are waiting for the cauliflower bits to get ready in the microwave, you may start preparing the onion.
3. Sauté chopped onions with 2 tablespoons of olive oil until browned, which should take around 5 minutes, then add garlic, nutmeg, and allspice to the pan. Stir in and cook for another 1 to 2 minutes, then add the cauliflower and egg substitute.
4. Stir in all ingredients to combine the mixture, then seal the pan and lower the heat. Cook for another 10 to 15 minutes, until cauliflower tortilla is browned. Serve by slicing the tortilla into 4 pieces.

Nutrition:
- Potassium: 272 mg
- Sodium: 148 mg
- Phosphorus: 78 mg
- Calories: 102

60. Eggs Benedict

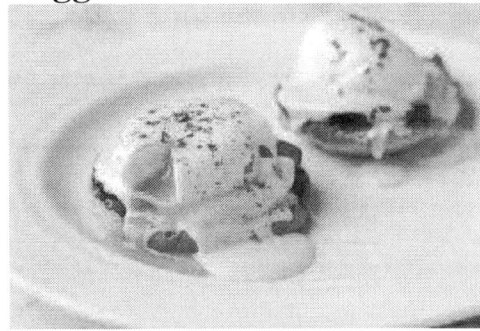

Preparation Time: 20 minutes
Cooking Time: 35 Minutes
Servings: 4
Ingredients:
- 2 pieces of toasted bread - white flour
- 4 eggs
- 3 egg yolks
- 1 tablespoon lemon juice
- ½ teaspoon of cayenne pepper
- ½ teaspoon of paprika
- 1 tablespoon apple cider vinegar
- 2 tablespoons of unsalted butter

Directions:
1. Slice the two toasted bread pieces in two, so you can end up with four pieces where each piece represents one serving.
2. Take a large skillet or a pot and pour one cup of water in it. Add a tablespoon of vinegar and bring the water to boil. When the water starts to boil, break four eggs, one at a time, and poach the eggs by covering the skillet. Eggs should be done between 3 and 5 minutes of poaching, depending on how you like your eggs cooked.
3. Next, place poached eggs on top of bread pieces. Take a skillet and add the butter to melt it, then add cayenne and paprika to the melted butter. Beat

the egg yolks over medium heat, then add the eggs to the mixture with butter. Add lemon juice and whisk it into the egg and butter mixture. Once the sauce reaches an adequate thickness, remove it from the heat and pour over the eggs and toasted bread.

Nutrition:
- Potassium: 146 mg
- Sodium: 206 mg
- Phosphorus: 114 mg
- Calories: 316

61. Cranberry and Apple Oatmeal

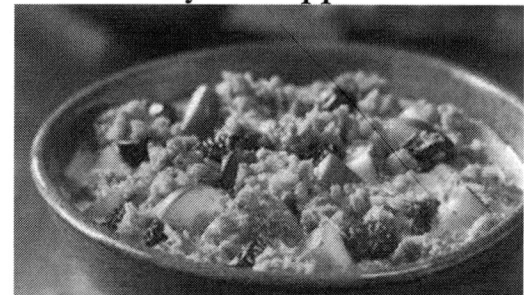

Preparation Time: 10 minutes
Cooking Time: 25 Minutes
Servings: 2
Ingredients:
- 1 apple – diced
- ¼ teaspoon nutmeg
- ¼ cup cranberry – fresh
- 2/3 cups of oatmeal – you can use quick oatmeal with no added sodium and extra potassium–avoid whole grain if not on dialysis
- ½ teaspoon cinnamon
- 2 cups of water

Directions:
1. You need to prepare all the ingredients and cut the apple into small pieces. Pour two cups of water into a saucepan and add the diced apple, cranberries, nutmeg, and cinnamon.
2. Seal the saucepan and bring the water with ingredients to boil. Cook until the fruit is tender, which shouldn't take more than 5 to 10 minutes.
3. Check if apples are tender, then add 2/3 cups oatmeal to the boiling water. Stir in and cook for around one minute before serving the oatmeal. Based on your doctor's recommendations you can serve the oatmeal with an adequate dose of milk or add milk substitute to the oatmeal when serving.

Nutrition:
- Potassium: 170 mg Sodium: 59 mg
- Phosphorus: 187 mg Calories: 173

62. Blueberry Breakfast Smoothie

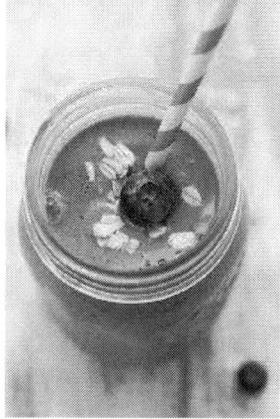

Preparation Time: 10 minutes
Cooking Time: 10 Minutes
Servings: 1
Ingredients:
- 1/3 cup vanilla almond milk – no sugar added
- 2 tablespoons protein powder of your choice

- ¼ cup of Greek yogurt - look for brands with low sodium and low potassium
- 3 strawberries - fresh, sliced
- 6 raspberries
- 1 cup blueberries – frozen or fresh
- 1 tablespoon cereal – avoid whole grain due to high levels of potassium

Directions:
1. First, you need to blend one cup of blueberries in a food processor, blending the fruit at low speed for around a minute.
2. After a minute, add almond milk, protein powder, and Greek yogurt to blended blueberries and blend the mixture for another minute or until the blueberry smoothie turns into a homogeneous mass.
3. Pour the smoothie into a bowl, add cereals, raspberries, sliced strawberries, and serve.

Nutrition:
- Potassium: 270 mg Sodium: 108 mg
- Phosphorus: 114 mg Calories: 225

63. Apple Sauce Cream Toast

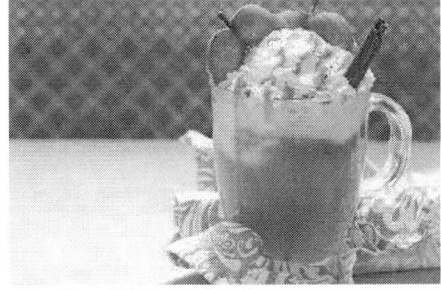

Preparation Time: 5 minutes
Cooking Time: 10 Minutes
Servings: 1
Ingredients:
- 2 tablespoons applesauce
- 2 slices of toast or white bread
- 1 egg white – uncooked, scrambled
- Cinnamon

Directions:
1. Whip the liquid uncooked egg white until foamy and take a skillet that doesn't stick. Heat the skillet, then soak one side of the toast into the egg white whip.
2. Bake the toast on the side where the toast is soaked into the egg white and while you are doing so, soak another piece of toast into the egg white whip and as you are baking the second toast piece, add applesauce on the second piece and seal with the first piece of toast once the outside crust is well baked.
3. Sprinkle with cinnamon to taste and serve.

Nutrition:
- Potassium: 294 mg
- Sodium: 366 mg
- Phosphorus: 158 mg
- Calories: 256

64. Waffles

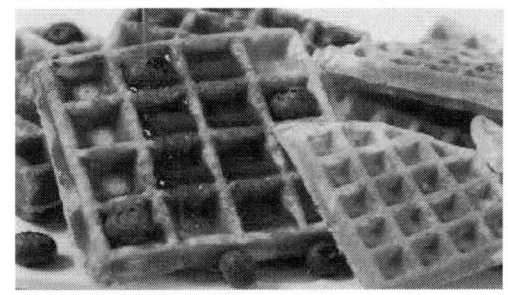

Preparation Time: 20 minutes
Cooking Time: 15 Minutes
Servings: 8
Ingredients:
- 1 ½ teaspoons yeast for baking
- 8 tablespoons butter – unsalted
- 2 eggs

- 1 ¾ cups of milk – 2% milkfat
- Sugar substitute to taste
- 1 teaspoon almond extract
- 2 cups flour – all-purpose

Directions:
1. Heat a saucepan and place the butter and milk in it. Wait for the butter to melt with occasional stirring. As you are waiting for the milk and butter mixture to cool off a bit so that the saucepan is warm to touch, you will take a bowl and whisk sugar substitute, yeast, and flour. Once combined, you will add the warm milk and butter mixture to the flour bowl and whisk some more until the mass is well combined.
2. Take another bowl and whisk the eggs with almond extract, adding the flour batter's whipped egg mixture. Stir in well to combine until you get a smooth, homogenous mass. The best option is to prepare the mixture a day ahead, as you will need to keep the dough in the fridge for at least 12 hours before baking.
3. Once you are ready to bake your waffles, you will set the oven to 200 degrees F and keep the waffle bowl near so that the dough is kept warm. Prepare your waffle maker and start making waffles by pouring the dough.

Nutrition:
- Potassium: 131 mg
- Sodium: 208 mg
- Phosphorus: 113 mg
- Calories: 223

65. Egg Whites and Veggie Bake

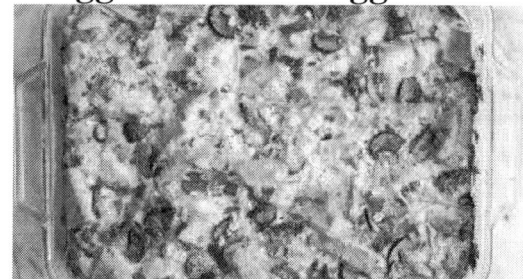

Preparation Time: 20 minutes
Cooking Time: 50 Minutes
Servings: 4
Ingredients:
- 1 cup broccoli florets
- 1 cup cauliflower florets
- 1 garlic clove - minced
- 6 egg whites – liquid, uncooked
- ½ cup bell pepper – diced
- 1 small onion – finely diced
- ½ cup low-sodium cheese

Directions:
1. Take care of the veggies, wash and dice the cauliflower, broccoli, and onion. While you are sautéing onion with a tablespoon of olive oil, place broccoli and cauliflower in a bowl with a tablespoon of water and place it in the microwave.
2. Microwave florets for 5 minutes before taking the bowl out of the microwave. The onions should be ready within 5 minutes when you should add the minced garlic and peppers. Sauté for another 3 to 4 minutes.
3. Combine broccoli and cauliflower florets with garlic, peppers, and onion, and let the veggie mixture cool off a bit as you are whisking egg whites. Egg whites should be whisked until foamy. Whisk in the cheese with the

egg whites, then add the veggie mixture to your egg whites, stirring the ingredients to combine it into a homogenous mass.
4. Take a medium baking dish and pour in the mixture. Preheat the oven to 350 degrees F and place the baking dish into the oven, baking the egg white veggie bake for 20 minutes or until the mixture settles.

Nutrition:
- Potassium: 163 mg
- Sodium: 89 mg
- Phosphorus: 105 mg
- Calories: 258

66. Peach Berry Parfait

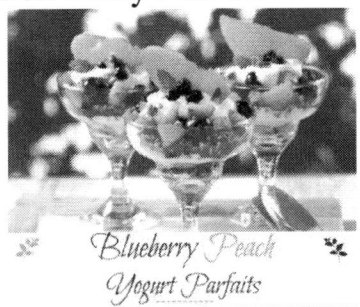

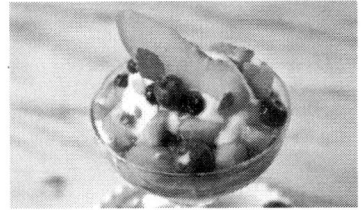

Preparation Time: 5 minutes
Cooking Time: 5 minutes
Servings: 2
Ingredients:
- 1 cup plain unsweetened yogurt, divided
- 1 teaspoon vanilla extract
- 1 small peach, diced
- ½ cup blueberries
- 2 tablespoons walnut pieces

Directions:
1. In a small bowl, combine the yogurt and vanilla.
2. Put 2 tablespoons of yogurt to each of 2 cups. Divide the diced peach and the blueberries between the cups, and top with the remaining yogurt.
3. Sprinkle each cup with 1 tablespoon of walnut pieces.

Nutrition:
- Calories: 191 Total Fat: 10 g
- Saturated Fat: 3 g
- Cholesterol: 15 mg
- Carbohydrates: 14 g
- Fiber: 14 g Protein: 12 g
- Phosphorus: 189 mg
- Potassium: 327 mg
- Sodium: 40 mg

67. Open-Faced Bagel Breakfast Sandwich

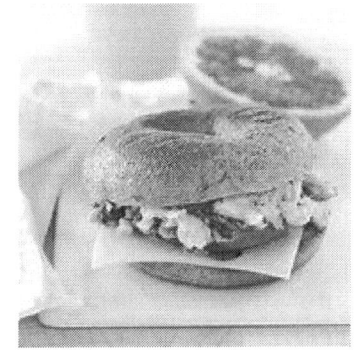

Preparation Time: 5 minutes
Cooking Time: 5 minutes
Servings: 2
Ingredients:
- 1 multigrain bagel, halved
- 2 slices tomato
- 1 slice red onion
- Freshly ground black pepper
- 1 cup microgreens

Directions:
1. Lightly toast the bagel.
2. Place the bagel halves, top each half with 1 slice of tomato and a couple of onion rings.
3. Season with black pepper. Top each half with ½ cup of microgreens and serve.

Nutrition:
- Calories: 156 Total Fat: 6 g
- Saturated Fat: 3 g
- Cholesterol: 18 mg
- Carbohydrates: 22 g Fiber: 3 g
- Protein: 5 g Protein: 5 g
- Phosphorus: 98 mg
- Potassium: 163 mg
- Sodium: 195 mg

68. Bulgur Bowl with Strawberries and Walnuts

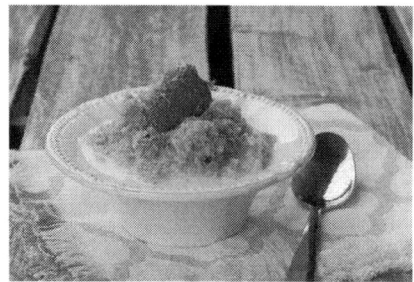

Preparation Time: 10 minutes
Cooking Time: 15 minutes
Servings: 4
Ingredients:
- 1 cup bulgur
- 1 cup strawberries, sliced
- 4 tablespoons (¼ cup) homemade rice milk or unsweetened store-bought rice milk
- 4 teaspoons brown sugar
- 4 teaspoons extra-virgin olive oil
- 4 tablespoons (¼ cup) walnut pieces
- 4 tablespoons (¼ cup) cacao nibs (optional)

Directions:
1. In a small pot, combine the bulgur with 2 cups of water. Bring to a boil, lower the heat and let simmer, covered, for 12 to 15 minutes, until tender.
2. In each of four bowls, add a quarter of the bulgur and top with ¼ cup of strawberries, 1 tablespoon of rice milk, 1 teaspoon of brown sugar, 1 teaspoon of olive oil, 1 tablespoon of walnut pieces, and 1 tablespoon of cacao nibs (if using).

Nutrition:
- Calories: 190 Total Fat: 9 g
- Saturated Fat: 1 g Cholesterol: 0 mg
- Carbohydrates: 26 g Fiber: 5 g
- Protein: 4 g Phosphorus: 66 mg
- Potassium: 153 mg Sodium: 13 mg

69. Overnight Oats Three Ways

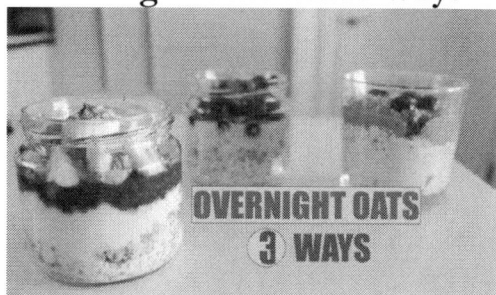

Preparation Time: 5 minutes
Cooking Time: 5 minutes
Servings: 2
Ingredients:
- ¾ cup homemade rice milk or unsweetened store-bought rice milk
- ½ cup plain unsweetened yogurt
- ½ cup rolled oats

- 1 tablespoon ground flaxseed
- 1 teaspoon vanilla extract
- 2 teaspoons honey

Directions:
1. In a medium bowl, mix the rice milk, yogurt, oats, flaxseed, vanilla, and honey.
2. Add the ingredients to make your preferred variation, and stir to blend.
3. Divide between two jars, cover, and refrigerate for at least 4 hours or overnight.

Nutrition:
- Calories: 196
- Total Fat: 7 g
- Saturated Fat: 2 g
- Cholesterol: 7 mg
- Carbohydrates: 25 g
- Fiber: 3 g
- Protein: 8 g
- Phosphorus: 99 mg
- Potassium: 114 mg
- Sodium: 63 mg

70. Buckwheat Pancakes

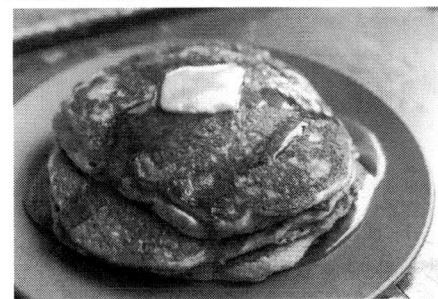

Preparation Time: 10 minutes
Cooking Time: 15 minutes
Servings: 4
Ingredients:
- 1¾ cups homemade rice milk or unsweetened store-bought rice milk
- 2 teaspoons white vinegar
- 1 cup buckwheat flour
- ½ cup all-purpose flour
- 1 tablespoon sugar
- 1 large egg
- 2 teaspoons Phosphorus-Free baking powder
- 1 teaspoon vanilla extract
- 2 tablespoons butter, for the skillet

Directions:
1. Combine the rice milk and vinegar. Let sit for 5 minutes.
2. Meanwhile, in a large bowl, mix the buckwheat flour and all-purpose flour. Add the sugar and baking powder, stirring to blend.
3. Add the egg and vanilla to the rice milk and stir to blend. Add the wet ingredients to the dry, and stir until just mixed.
4. Melt 1½ teaspoons of butter. Use a ¼-cup measuring cup to scoop the batter into the skillet. Cook for 2 to 3 minutes, until small bubbles form on the surface of the pancakes. Flip and cook on the opposite side for 1 to 2 minutes.
5. Transfer the pancakes to a serving platter, and in batches, continue cooking the remaining batter in the skillet, adding more butter as needed.

Nutrition:
- Calories: 264 Total Fat: 9 g
- Saturated Fat: 3 g
- Cholesterol: 58 mg
- Carbohydrates: 39 g
- Fiber: 3 g Protein: 7 g
- Phosphorus: 147 mg
- Potassium: 399 mg
- Sodium: 232 mg

71. Broccoli Basil Quiche

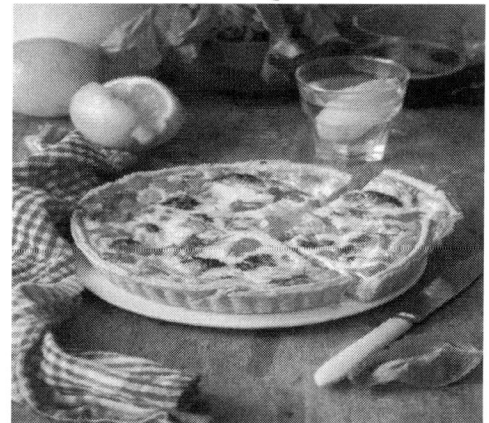

Preparation Time: 10 minutes
Cooking Time: 55 minutes
Servings: 8
Ingredients:

- 1 store-bought frozen piecrust
- 2 cups finely chopped broccoli
- 1 tomato, chopped
- 2 scallions, chopped
- 3 eggs, beaten
- 2 tablespoons chopped basil
- 1 cup homemade rice milk or unsweetened store-bought rice milk
- ½ cup crumbled feta cheese
- 1 garlic clove, minced
- 1 tablespoon all-purpose flour
- Freshly ground black pepper

Directions:
1. Preheat the oven to 425°F.
2. Line a pie pan with the piecrust, and use a fork to pierce the crust in several places. Bake the crust for 10 minutes. Remove from the oven and reduce the temperature to 325°F.
3. In a medium bowl, mix the broccoli, tomato, scallions, eggs, basil, rice milk, feta, garlic, and flour. Season with pepper.
4. Pour the broccoli-and-egg mixture into the prepared pie pan. Bake for 35 to 45 minutes, until a knife inserted in the center comes out clean. Let cool for 10 to 15 minutes before serving.

Nutrition:
- Calories: 160
- Total Fat: 10 g
- Saturated Fat: 3 g
- Cholesterol: 87 mg
- Carbohydrates: 13 g
- Fiber: 1 g
- Protein: 6 g
- Phosphorus: 101 mg
- Potassium: 173 mg
- Sodium: 259 mg

72. Poor Knight with Apple Compote

Preparation Time: 15 minutes
Cooking Time: 0 minutes
Servings: 4
Ingredients:

- 4 large (or 8 small) slices of white bread
- 80 ml of cream
- 120ml water
- 1 egg
- 1 teaspoon vanilla pudding powder (for cooking)
- 2 tbsp sugar
- Breadcrumbs
- 40 g butter
- Sugar and cinnamon to taste
- 400 g apple compote

Directions:
1. Mix the cream and water and stir together with the pudding powder, sugar, and egg until smooth. Halve or

quarter the white bread slices and turn in the egg mixture.
2. Then turn in breadcrumbs and bake in hot butter over mild heat until golden brown on both sides.
3. Sprinkle with cinnamon sugar to taste and serve with the apple compote.

Nutrition:
- Calories: 416
- Protein: 7 g
- Potassium: 192 mg
- Sodium: 185 mg

73. Papaya and Cranberry Jam
Preparation Time: 8 minutes
Cooking Time: 10 minutes
Servings: 6
Ingredients:
- Pulp of a ripe papaya 700 grams
- Lemon juice 4 tbsp
- Cranberries / Cranberries 100 grams
- Preserving sugar 1: 1 1000 grams

Directions:
1. With hot water, wash the papayas, rub them dry and peel them. Then cut it in half with a teaspoon and scrape the seeds out. With the lemon juice, purée the pulp. The cranberries are washed and sorted, put in a large saucepan, and lightly mashed with a fork. Add the papaya fruit puree and 1:1 of the gelling sugar and mix well.
2. While stirring, bring to the boil over high heat until all the food bubbles vigorously. Now the time for cooking begins! Let it simmer for 4 minutes, constantly stirring.
3. Remove the pot from the stove. Fill the hot mass quickly with jars rinsed with hot water to the brim and close immediately with the screw cap.

Nutrition:
- Calories: 344
- Protein: 0.1 g
- Potassium: 31 mg
- Sodium: 182 mg

74. Lemon Curd
Preparation Time: 5 minutes
Cooking Time: 75 minutes
Servings: 6
Ingredients:
- Freshly squeezed lemon juice 150 ml
- Freshly squeezed orange juice 100 ml
- Butter 100 gr.
- Sifted corn starch 30 gr.
- White wine dry 150 ml
- Sugar 150 gr.
- Grated lemon peel 1 pc.

Directions:
1. Melt the butter and heat the cornstarch while stirring until it is light yellow. Add lemon and orange juice and the white wine. Please make sure that there are no lumps.
2. Now add the sugar and lemon zest and let it cook for another 2 minutes. Fill everything into glasses immediately.
3. The lemon curd unfortunately only lasts about 3 days in the refrigerator.

Nutrition:
- Calories: 239
- Protein: 0.3 g
- Potassium: 28 mg
- Sodium: 171 mg

75. Pancakes with Raspberries and Ricotta

Preparation Time: 21 minutes
Cooking Time: 32 minutes
Servings: 2
Ingredients:
- 100 g flour
- 1 egg
- 200 ml of mineral water
- 50ml cream
- 1 tsp baking soda
- 1 pinch of salt
- 2 tbsp rapeseed oil
- 80 g raspberries
- 2 tbsp liquid honey
- 200 g ricotta

Directions:
1. Mix the flour with the egg, mineral water, cream, salt, and baking powder.
2. Let the dough rest for 10 minutes and fry 2 pancakes in hot rapeseed oil.
3. Fill with ricotta and raspberries and pour the honey over them.

Nutrition:
- Calories: 574
- Protein: 21 g
- Potassium: 294 mg
- Sodium: 112 mg

76. Muesli Made From Rice Flakes

Preparation Time: 8 minutes
Cooking Time: 10 minutes
Servings: 2
Ingredients:
- 50 ml of cream
- 150 ml of water
- 2 tbsp sugar
- 35 g rice flakes
- 50 g blueberries from the glass, drained
- Fresh mint

Directions:
1. Bring the cream and water to the boil in a saucepan, then add the rice flakes and sugar, bring to the boil again briefly and remove from the stove. Let it soak for 10 minutes.
2. Divide between 2 bowls, add blueberries, and serve with the mint.

Nutrition:
- Calories: 200
- Protein: 2 g
- Potassium: 68 mg
- Sodium: 10 mg

77. Muesli Mix

Preparation Time: 11 minutes
Cooking Time: 16 minutes
Servings: 4
Ingredients:
- 200 g millet flakes
- 150 g corn flakes
- 150 g rice crisps or puffed rice
- 50 g desiccated coconut
- 50 g sugar

Directions:
1. Brown the coconut flakes with the sugar in a pan. Let cool and mix in the other ingredients. Store in a sealable jar.
2. Serve with a cream/water mixture and fruit compote (without juice) or quark.

Nutrition:
- Calories: 231 Protein: 4 g
- Potassium: 67 mg
- Sodium: 117 mg

78. Bamboo Bread (Low Carb)
Preparation Time: 7 minutes
Cooking Time: 41 minutes
Servings: 2
Ingredients:
- 150 g onions
- 1 tbsp olive oil
- 250 g low-fat quark
- 2 eggs
- 80 g of oat bran
- 25 g bamboo fibbers
- 30 g de-oiled gold flaxseed flour
- 1 teaspoon of tartar baking powder
- 1 teaspoon salt

Directions:
1. Preheat the oven to 175 degrees (convection).
2. Peel the onions and cut them into cubes. Cook oil in a pan and gently fry the onion cubes for 5 to 6 minutes.
3. Then mix the onions well with all the other ingredients in a mixing bowl. Butter a rectangular baking pan or line it with baking paper.
4. Pour in the batter and bake for 30-35 minutes. Let cool well before turning over.

Nutrition:
- Calories: 344
- Protein: 5 g
- Potassium: 23 mg
- Sodium: 189 mg

79. Open Bread with Avocado
Preparation Time: 13 minutes
Cooking Time: 0 minutes
Servings: 2
Ingredients
- ½ avocado
- To taste: lemon juice
- 1 slice (40 g, e.g., spelled and rye) whole grain bread
- 200 g vegetables
- Salt
- Pepper

Directions:
1. Peel the avocado and remove the seed. Drizzle the pulp with a little lemon juice, if you like, and either put it in fine slices on the wholemeal bread or mash with a fork and spread on the bread. Season with a little salt and pepper (fresh from the mill).
2. Wash the vegetables (for example, some tomatoes, cucumber, paprika, and carrots), cut into small pieces, and serve as a raw vegetable side dish with bread.

Nutrition:
- Calories: 304
- Protein: 10 g
- Potassium: 13 mg
- Sodium: 91 mg

80. Bircher Muesli with Papaya
Preparation Time: 5 minutes
Cooking Time: 0 minutes
Servings: 2
Ingredients:
- 80 g crispy oat flakes
- 1 tbsp raisins
- ¼ l (1.5% fat) milk
- alternatively: ¼ l water
- 1 small (approx. 300 g) papaya
- 1 apple
- 150 g (1.5% fat) natural yogurt
- 2 teaspoons of lemon juice
- 1 tbsp pecan nuts
- 1 tbsp dried apple chips

Directions:
1. Mix the oat flakes and raisins in a bowl with the milk (in the case of kidney stones, with water) the day before and leave to soak in the refrigerator for about 12 hours, preferably overnight.
2. The next day, cut the papaya in half, remove the core, peel and cut the pulp into 1-2 cm cubes. Wash the apple and grate finely around the core on a vegetable grater. Stir grated apple and half of the papaya cubes with the yogurt into the oatmeal mix. Finally, add the lemon juice to taste.
3. Spread the muesli mix on bowls. Roughly chop the pecans (omit if there are kidney stones) and sprinkle with the rest of the papaya. Serve garnished with the apple chips.

Nutrition:
- Calories: 420
- Protein: 11 g
- Potassium: 30 mg
- Sodium: 171 mg

81. Cauliflower and Broccoli Curry
Preparation Time: 9 minutes
Cooking Time: 22 minutes
Servings: 2
Ingredients:
- 100 g chicken breast fillet
- 100 g cauliflower
- 100 g broccoli
- 1 tbsp rapeseed oil
- 1 tbsp curry powder
- 100 ml vegetable broth
- 100 ml coconut milk

Directions:
1. Wash the meat, pat it dry and dice it. The vegetables should be washed and cleaned and cut into small florets. Instead of being fresh, frozen vegetables can also be used.
2. In a bigger pan, heat the oil, fry the meat cubes for approximately 2 minutes and add the vegetables. Briefly fry and stir in the powder with the curry. Stir in coconut milk and vegetable stock, and simmer for 8-10 minutes. Put a bit of salt to taste if necessary.

Nutrition:
- Calories: 463
- Protein: 30 g
- Potassium: 21 mg
- Sodium: 151 mg

82. Broccoli and Lentil Salad with Mackerel
Preparation Time: 10 minutes
Cooking Time: 12 minutes
Servings: 2
Ingredients:
- 300 g broccoli
- 1 small onion
- 4 tbsp orange juice
- 2 tbsp white wine vinegar
- 2 tbsp olive oil
- Salt
- From the mill: pepper
- 1 teaspoon (from the jar) grated horseradish
- 1 can (240 g drained weight) lentils
- 125 g of cocktail tomatoes
- 4 stalks of basil
- 2 smoked (approx. 150 g, skin-on) mackerel fillets

Directions:
1. Wash and cut the broccoli into florets, peel the stalks and cut into small cubes. Peel the onion and cut it into fine cubes.
2. In a small saucepan, bring the onion cubes to the boil with orange juice, vinegar, and olive oil. Add the broccoli and cook covered over medium heat for about 3 minutes. Pull away from heat and sprinkle with salt, pepper, and horseradish.
3. Rinse the lentils in a sieve and let them drain well. Wash and halve the tomatoes. Gently mix the lentils and tomatoes into the broccoli.
4. Wash the basil, pat dry, and pluck the leaves. Peel the mackerel fillets and cut them into bite-sized pieces. Cover the salad with the mackerel pieces, sprinkle with basil, and season with pepper.

Nutrition:
- Calories: 380
- Protein: 17 g
- Potassium: 27 mg
- Sodium: 122 mg

83. Broccoli Rice Gratin (Italian Style)

Preparation Time: 30 minutes
Cooking Time: 47 minutes
Servings: 2
Ingredients:
- 125 g (10-minute rice
- Salt
- 300 g broccoli florets
- Salt
- From the mill: pepper
- 1 teaspoon dried Italian herb
- 1 teaspoon (noble sweet variety) paprika powder
- 125 g (8.5% fat) small mozzarella balls
- 2 tbsp pine nuts
- Some basil leaves

Directions:
1. Following the directions on the packet, cook the rice with plenty of salted water. Meanwhile, clean the broccoli florets and wash them, and cut them into smaller pieces. Add the broccoli to the rice about 5 minutes before cooking time ends, bring it all to a boil again, and simultaneously cook the broccoli.
2. Set the oven to 220 ° C. Brush baking dish (20 x 30 cm approx.) with oil. Drain in a colander with the rice and broccoli and drain. Use salt, pepper, Italian herbs, and paprika powder to season the tomatoes. Mix and dissolve in the baking dish with the broccoli rice mix.
3. Rinse and chop cherry tomatoes in half. Halve the balls of mozzarella as well. Combine the tomatoes and mozzarella, sprinkle with the pine nuts, and spread on the broccoli-rice mix. On the middle rack, bake the gratin in the oven for about 10 minutes. To serve, sprinkle with the basil leaves.

Nutrition:
- Calories: 320
- Protein: 18 g
- Potassium: 45 mg
- Sodium: 142 mg

84. Colorful Bean Salad

Preparation Time: 11 minutes
Cooking Time: 0 minutes
Servings: 4

Ingredients:
- 200 g green beans
- 1 onion
- 1 bell pepper
- 1 small can (drained weight 250 g) white beans
- 1 small can (drained weight 250 g) kidney beans
- 2 tbsp wine vinegar
- 2 tbsp sour cream
- ½ teaspoon mustard
- ½ teaspoon tomato ketchup
- ½ teaspoon horseradish
- Salt
- Pepper
- 1 tbsp oil
- Chopped thyme

Directions:
1. Clean and wash the green beans and cook in salted boiling water for 6-8 minutes until they are firm to the bite. Pour into a sieve, rinse in cold water and drain well. Transfer to a large bowl.
2. Skin the onion and cut it into thin rings. Halve and core the peppers lengthways, wash and cut into cubes. Drain the kidney beans and white beans each into a sieve, rinse with cold water and drain well. Then add the onion, bell pepper, kidney beans, and white beans to the green beans.
3. For the dressing, mix together vinegar, sour cream, mustard, tomato ketchup, horseradish, oil, and thyme, season with salt and pepper. Mix with the salad ingredients and let the bean salad steep for about 5 minutes before serving.

Nutrition:
- Calories: 210
- Protein: 7 g
- Potassium: 29 mg
- Sodium: 132 mg

CHAPTER 4:

Main Dishes

85. Corn and Shrimp Quiche

Preparation Time: 15 minutes
Cooking Time: 50 minutes
Servings: 6
Ingredients:
- 1 cup small cooked shrimp
- 1½ cups frozen corn, thawed and drained
- 5 large eggs, beaten
- 1 cup unsweetened almond milk
- Pinch salt
- ⅛ teaspoon freshly ground black pepper

Directions:
1. Preheat the oven to 350°F. Spray a 9-inch pie pan with nonstick baking spray.
2. In the prepared pan, combine the shrimp and corn.
3. In a medium bowl, beat the eggs, almond milk, salt, and pepper. Gently pour into the pan.
4. Bake for 45 to 55 minutes or until the quiche is puffed, set to the touch, and light golden brown on top. Let stand for 10 minutes before cutting into wedges to serve.

Ingredient Tip: Shrimp are measured according to the number per pound. So bigger shrimp have a lower number per pound. For this recipe, small shrimp should be about 50 per pound. Medium shrimp are usually 36 to 40 per pound. You can cut larger shrimp into small pieces instead of buying small shrimp if you'd like.

Nutrition:
- Calories: 198
- Total Fat: 10 g
- Saturated Fat: 4 g
- Sodium: 238 mg
- Phosphorus: 260 mg
- Potassium: 261 mg
- Carbohydrates: 9 g
- Fiber: 1 g
- Protein: 20 g
- Sugar: 2 g

86. Ginger-Orange Tuna Pasta Salad

Preparation Time: 20 minutes
Cooking Time: 9 minutes
Servings: 6
Ingredients:
- 3 cups whole-wheat ziti pasta
- 1 large navel orange, zested and juiced
- ¼ cup extra-virgin olive oil
- 2 tablespoons yellow prepared mustard
- ¼ teaspoon ground ginger
- Pinch salt
- 1 large navel orange, peeled and segmented
- 1 (6-ounce) can light low-sodium tuna, drained

Directions:
1. Bring a large pot of water to a boil. Add the pasta and cook according to package directions until the pasta is al dente. Drain and set aside.
2. In a large bowl, whisk the orange juice and zest, olive oil, mustard, ginger, and salt until combined. Add the orange segments and tuna and stir to coat.
3. When the pasta is done, drain and add to the bowl with the dressing and other ingredients. Toss to coat.
4. Cover and chill the salad for 2 to 3 hours, stirring once.

Increase Protein Tip: To make this a medium-protein recipe, add one more can of drained tuna. The protein content will increase to 19 g per serving.

Nutrition:
- Calories: 305 Total Fat: 11 g
- Saturated Fat: 2 g Sodium: 105 mg
- Phosphorus: 218 mg
- Potassium: 379 mg
- Carbohydrates: 43 g
- Fiber: 6 g Protein: 13 g
- Sugar: 7 g

87. Pineapple-Soy Salmon Stir-Fry

Preparation Time: 15 minutes
Cooking Time: 15 minutes
Servings: 4
Ingredients:
- 1 (8-ounce) can crushed pineapple, strained, reserving juice
- 2 tablespoons low-sodium soy sauce
- 1 tablespoon cornstarch
- ⅛ teaspoon freshly ground black pepper
- 2 tablespoons extra-virgin olive oil
- 2 (6-ounce) salmon fillets without skin, cubed
- 1 (16-ounce) bag frozen stir-fry vegetables

Directions:
1. In a small bowl, whisk the reserved pineapple juice, soy sauce, cornstarch, and pepper and set aside.
2. In a large wok or skillet, heat the olive oil. Add the salmon cubes and stir-fry for 3 to 4 minutes, or until the salmon flakes with a fork. Using a slotted spoon, transfer the salmon to a plate and set aside.
3. Add the frozen vegetables to the wok and stir-fry for another 3 to 4 minutes, or until the vegetables are hot and tender.
4. Return the salmon to the wok and add the pineapple.
5. Whisk the sauce again and add to the wok; stir-fry for 3 to 4 minutes or until the sauce bubbles and has thickened. Serve.

Ingredient Tip: You can make this recipe with just about any protein, such as cubed boneless skinless chicken breasts, cod or sole, or peeled and deveined shrimp. To make this recipe gluten-free, use low-sodium tamari instead of soy sauce.

Nutrition:
- Calories: 280
- Total Fat: 13 g
- Saturated Fat: 2 g
- Sodium: 361 mg
- Phosphorus: 271 mg
- Potassium: 599 mg
- Carbohydrates: 21 g
- Fiber: 3 g Protein: 22 g
- Sugar: 11 g

88. Fish Taco Filling

Preparation Time: 15 minutes
Cooking Time: 10 minutes
Servings: 4
Ingredients:
- 2 tablespoons extra-virgin olive oil
- 2 shallots, minced
- 3 (6-ounce) sole fillets, cut into strips
- 2 teaspoons chili powder
- 1 lime, zested and juiced
- 3 cups cabbage coleslaw mix with carrots

Directions:
1. In a large skillet, heat the olive oil over medium heat.
2. Add the shallots and cook for 3 minutes, stirring, until softened.
3. Add the sole fillets and sprinkle with the chili powder. Cook for 3 to 5 minutes, stirring gently, until the fish flakes when tested with a fork. Remove the skillet from the heat.
4. Drizzle the lime zest and juice over the fish.
5. Serve with the coleslaw in tacos or over rice.

Increase Protein Tip: To make this a medium-protein recipe, add one more 6-ounce sole fillet. The protein content will increase to 18 g per servings.

Ingredient Tip: If you like spicy food, you can add 1 diced medium jalapeño pepper to the shallots or add ½ teaspoon of red pepper flakes to the fish mixture along with the lime juice and zest.

Nutrition:
- Calories: 176
- Total Fat: 9 g
- Saturated Fat: 1 g
- Sodium: 315 mg
- Phosphorus: 265 mg
- Potassium: 451 mg
- Carbohydrates: 14 g
- Fiber: 4 g
- Protein: 13 g
- Sugar: 6 g

89. Ginger Shrimp with Snow Peas

Preparation Time: 20 minutes
Cooking Time: 12 minutes
Servings: 4
Ingredients:
- 2 tablespoons extra-virgin olive oil
- 1 tablespoon minced peeled fresh ginger
- 2 cups snow peas
- 1½ cups frozen baby peas
- 3 tablespoons water
- 1-pound medium shrimp, shelled and deveined
- 2 tablespoons low-sodium soy sauce
- ⅛ teaspoon freshly ground black pepper

Directions:
1. In a large wok or skillet, heat the olive oil over medium heat.
2. Add the ginger and stir-fry for 1 to 2 minutes, until the ginger is fragrant.
3. Add the snow peas and stir-fry for 2 to 3 minutes, until they are tender-crisp.
4. Add the baby peas and the water and stir. Cover the wok and steam for 2 to 3 minutes or until the vegetables are tender.
5. Stir in the shrimp and stir-fry for 3 to 4 minutes, or until the shrimp have curled and turned pink.
6. Add the soy sauce and pepper; stir and serve.

Ingredient Tip: Snow peas can have a tough string along one side that won't soften very well during the stir-fry process. Just pinch the curly end of the pod and pull to remove it. Discard the string.

Nutrition:
- Calories: 237
- Total Fat: 7 g
- Saturated Fat: 1 g
- Sodium: 469 mg
- Phosphorus: 350 mg
- Potassium: 504 mg
- Carbohydrates: 12 g
- Fiber: 4 g
- Protein: 32 g
- Sugar: 5 g

90. Roasted Cod with Plums
Preparation Time: 10 minutes
Cooking Time: 20 minutes
Servings: 4
Ingredients:
- 6 red plums, halved and pitted
- 1½ pounds cod fillets
- 3 tablespoons extra-virgin olive oil
- 2 tablespoons freshly squeezed lemon juice
- ½ teaspoon dried thyme leaves
- ⅛ teaspoon salt
- ⅛ teaspoon freshly ground black pepper
- ¾ cup plain whole-milk yogurt, for servings

Directions:
1. Preheat the oven to 375°F. Line a baking sheet with parchment paper.
2. Arrange the plums, cut-side up, along with the fish on the prepared baking sheet. Drizzle with the olive oil and lemon juice and sprinkle with the thyme, salt, and pepper.
3. Roast for 15 to 20 minutes or until the fish flakes when tested with a fork and the plums are tender.
4. Serve with the yogurt.

Ingredient Tip: There's no need to measure out exactly 2 tablespoons of lemon juice. A standard-size lemon has approximately 2 tablespoons of juice in it. Simply squeeze all the juice from the lemon, being careful to avoid squeezing in the seeds.

Nutrition:
- Calories: 230
- Total Fat: 9 g
- Saturated Fat: 2 g
- Sodium: 154 mg
- Phosphorus: 197 mg
- Potassium: 437 mg
- Carbohydrates: 10 g
- Fiber: 1 g
- Protein: 27 g
- Sugar: 8 g

91. Lemon Chicken
Preparation Time: 20 minutes
Cooking Time: 24 minutes
Servings: 4
Ingredients:
- 2 lemons
- 12 ounces' boneless skinless chicken breasts, cubed
- 2 tablespoons extra-virgin olive oil
- ⅛ teaspoon salt
- ⅛ teaspoon freshly ground black pepper
- ½ large onion, chopped
- 1 cup 2-inch green bean pieces
- 1 cup 2-inch asparagus pieces

Directions:

1. Zest one of the lemons and place the zest into a medium bowl. Juice that lemon and add the juice to the bowl. Slice the remaining lemon, remove the seeds, and set aside.
2. In the bowl with the lemon juice, place the cubed chicken and set aside for 10 minutes to marinate.
3. When ready to cook, in a large skillet, heat the olive oil over medium heat.
4. Using a slotted spoon, remove the chicken from the lemon juice, reserving the lemon juice mixture. Add the chicken to the pan and cook for 3 to 4 minutes, stirring, until the chicken is lightly browned. It doesn't have to be completely cooked. Transfer the chicken to a clean plate and sprinkle with salt and pepper.
5. Add the sliced lemon to the skillet and cook for 3 minutes on each side, turning once, until it is slightly caramelized. Transfer to the plate with the chicken.
6. Add the onion to the skillet and cook for 3 to 4 minutes, until the onion is tender-crisp, stirring to loosen the chicken drippings from the skillet.
7. Add the green beans and sauté for 2 minutes. Add the asparagus and sauté for 1 minute. Return the chicken to the skillet and add the reserved lemon juice. Simmer for 4 to 6 minutes or until the chicken is thoroughly cooked to 165°F, the vegetables are tender, and the sauce has slightly thickened.
8. Add the caramelized lemon slices to the skillet and cook for 1 to 2 minutes, stirring, until hot. Serve.

Nutrition:

- Calories: 207
- Total Fat: 9 g
- Saturated Fat: 1 g
- Sodium: 121 mg
- Phosphorus: 245 mg
- Potassium: 593 mg
- Carbohydrates: 11 g
- Fiber: 4 g
- Protein: 22 g
- Sugar: 5 g

92. Curried Chicken Stir-Fry

Preparation Time: 20 minutes
Cooking Time: 15 minutes
Servings: 6
Ingredients:

- 12 ounces' boneless skinless chicken breasts, cut into 1-inch cubes
- 2 teaspoons curry powder
- ⅛ teaspoon salt
- ⅛ teaspoon freshly ground black pepper
- 1 (20-ounce) can pineapple tidbits, strained, reserving juice
- 2 tablespoons extra-virgin olive oil
- 1 yellow onion, chopped
- 2 red bell peppers, chopped

Directions:

1. In a medium bowl, toss the chicken, curry powder, salt, and pepper and set aside.
2. In a small saucepan, heat the reserved pineapple juice over low heat. Let it reduce, occasionally stirring while you make the rest of the stir-fry.
3. In a large skillet, heat the olive oil over medium heat. Add the chicken. Stir-fry for 3 for 4 minutes or until the chicken is light brown; it doesn't have

to cook completely. Transfer the chicken to a plate.
4. Add the onion to the skillet and cook for 3 minutes, stirring, until the onion is crisp-tender. Check to make sure the pineapple liquid isn't burning and continue to stir it. Add the bell peppers and stir-fry for another 3 minutes, until crisp-tender.
5. Return the chicken to the skillet, add the pineapple tidbits and cook, stirring, for 3 to 4 minutes or until the chicken is cooked through.
6. Add the thickened pineapple juice to the skillet and stir. Serve.

Increase Protein Tip: To make this a high-protein recipe, increase the chicken to 1 pound. The protein content will increase to 25 g per servings.

Nutrition:
- Calories: 215
- Total Fat: 7 g
- Saturated Fat: 1 g
- Sodium: 98 mg
- Phosphorus: 146 mg
- Potassium: 374 mg
- Carbohydrates: 19 g
- Fiber: 2 g
- Protein: 19 g
- Sugar: 16 g

93. Thai-Style Chicken Salad
Preparation Time: 15 minutes
Cooking Time: 10 minutes
Servings: 6
Ingredients:
- 3 cups shredded cooked chicken (about 1 pound)
- 1 (10-ounce) package shredded cabbage with carrots
- 2 limes
- ⅓ cup extra-virgin olive oil
- ¼ cup peanut butter
- ¼ teaspoon freshly ground black pepper
- ¼ cup chopped peanuts

Directions:
1. In a large bowl, combine the chicken and cabbage and toss to mix.
2. In a small bowl, zest one of the limes. Juice both of the limes into the bowl. Add the olive oil, peanut butter, and pepper and mix with a whisk.
3. Drizzle the dressing over the salad and toss. Top with the peanuts and serve.

Ingredient Tip: If you like spicy food, add 1 or 2 minced jalapeño peppers to this salad. You could also add minced chipotle peppers in adobo sauce; just a teaspoon of each will add lots of heat.

Nutrition:
- Calories: 415
- Total Fat: 31 g
- Saturated Fat: 5 g
- Sodium: 119 mg
- Phosphorus: 239 mg
- Potassium: 408 mg
- Carbohydrates: 9 g
- Fiber: 3 g
- Protein: 28 g
- Sugar: 3 g

94. Chicken Casserole
Preparation Time: 30 minutes
Cooking Time: 75 minutes
Servings: 6
Ingredients:
- 2 tablespoons extra-virgin olive oil
- 6 bone-in skin-on chicken thighs

- 1 yellow onion, chopped
- 2½ cups plus ⅓ cup water
- ¼ teaspoon salt
- 3 cups frozen mixed vegetables
- 3 tablespoons flour
- ⅛ teaspoon freshly ground black pepper
- 1 cup crushed crisp rice cereal

Directions:
1. In a large saucepan, heat the olive oil over medium heat.
2. Add the chicken thighs, skin-side down. Brown the skin thoroughly, moving the chicken around from time to time when it no longer sticks to the pan. This should take 12 to 15 minutes.
3. Remove the chicken from the skillet. Add the onion; cook and stir for 2 minutes to loosen the pan drippings.
4. Return the chicken to the skillet and add 2½ cups of water and salt. Bring to a simmer, then reduce the heat to low and simmer for 30 to 40 minutes, occasionally stirring until the chicken reaches 165°F and the juices run clear.
5. Remove the chicken from the saucepan and let cool for 10 minutes while keeping the broth simmering. Then remove the meat from the skin and bones. Discard the skin and bones; shred the meat and return to the saucepan.
6. Add the frozen vegetables and bring to a simmer. Simmer for 3 to 5 minutes, stirring occasionally, or until the vegetables are thawed.
7. Combine the flour with the remaining ⅓ cup of water and pepper; mix well. Stir into the saucepan and simmer for 3 to 5 minutes or until the sauce has thickened.
8. Preheat the oven to 400°F.
9. Pour the chicken mixture into a 2-quart baking dish and top with the cereal.
10. Bake for 20 to 25 minutes, or until the filling is bubbling and the cereal is lightly browned. Serve.

Increase Protein Tip: To make this a high-protein recipe, use 8 bone-in, skin-on chicken thighs. The protein content will increase to 28 grams per serving.

Nutrition:
- Calories: 203
- Total Fat: 9 g
- Saturated Fat: 2 g
- Sodium: 181 mg
- Phosphorus: 178 mg
- Potassium: 264 mg
- Carbohydrates: 9 g
- Fiber: 2 g
- Protein: 21 g
- Sugar: 1 g

95. Chicken Patties with Dill

Preparation Time: 25 minutes
Cooking Time: 20 minutes
Servings: 4
Ingredients:
- 3 tablespoons extra-virgin olive oil, divided
- 1 large carrot, finely grated or diced
- 1 yellow onion, grated or diced
- ½ cup puffed rice cereal, crushed
- 1 teaspoon dried dill weed
- Pinch salt
- ⅛ teaspoon freshly ground black pepper
- 1-pound lean ground chicken

Directions:
1. In a large skillet, heat 1 tablespoon of olive oil over medium heat.
2. Add the carrot and onion and cook for 4 to 6 minutes, until tender. Add the crushed cereal, dill, salt, and pepper and stir. Transfer the vegetable mixture into a medium bowl and let cool for 15 minutes. Do not wipe out or wash the skillet.
3. Add the ground chicken to the vegetables and work gently but thoroughly with your hands until combined.
4. Form the chicken mixture into 4 patties, place onto a plate, and freeze for 10 minutes, so they firm up and are easier to work with.
5. In the same skillet, heat the remaining 2 tablespoons of olive oil over medium heat. Add the chicken patties; cook for 6 to 7 minutes per side, turning once, until the patties reach 165°F and the juices run clear. Serve.

Nutrition:
- Calories: 311 Total Fat: 15 g
- Saturated Fat: 3 g Sodium: 140 mg
- Phosphorus: 262 mg
- Potassium: 389 mg
- Carbohydrates: 6 g
- Fiber: 1 g Protein: 36 g
- Sugar: 2 g

96. Chicken and Cabbage Stir-Fry
Preparation Time: 25 minutes
Cooking Time: 20 minutes
Servings: 4
Ingredients:
- 2 tablespoons extra-virgin olive oil
- 8 ounces' boneless skinless chicken breasts, cubed
- 1 yellow onion, chopped
- 1 red bell pepper, chopped
- 1 (16-ounce) package cabbage coleslaw blend with carrots
- ⅓ cup water
- 2 tablespoons low-sodium soy sauce

Directions:
1. In a large skillet, heat the olive oil over medium heat.
2. Add the chicken and stir-fry for 5 to 6 minutes, or until the chicken is cooked through. Transfer the chicken to a plate and set aside.
3. Add the onion to the skillet and stir-fry for 3 to 4 minutes, or until crisp-tender, scraping the pan to loosen any bits.
4. Add the bell pepper and stir-fry for another 2 minutes, until crisp-tender.
5. Add the coleslaw mix and stir-fry for 3 to 5 minutes longer, until softened.
6. Return the chicken to the skillet along with the water and soy sauce and stir-fry for 3 to 5 minutes longer, or until the sauce is slightly thickened and the vegetables are tender. Serve.

Increase Protein Tip: To make this a high-protein recipe, only use half of the coleslaw blend and increase the chicken to ¾ pound. The protein content will increase to 28 g per servings.

Nutrition:
- Calories: 206 Total Fat: 9 g
- Saturated Fat: 2 g
- Sodium: 413 mg
- Phosphorus: 173 mg
- Potassium: 621 mg
- Carbohydrates: 13 g Fiber: 4 g
- Protein: 20 g
- Sugar: 6 g

97. Slow Cooker Chicken with Apple and Onions

Preparation Time: 15 minutes
Cooking Time: 6 hours
Servings: 4
Ingredients:
- 1 large yellow onion, chopped
- 6 boneless skinless chicken thighs, cut into strips
- 3 Granny Smith apples, sliced
- 2 tablespoons Dijon mustard
- 2 tablespoons honey
- 1/8 teaspoon salt
- 1/8 teaspoon freshly ground black pepper

Directions:
1. In a 4 or 5-quart slow cooker, place the onions. Top with the chicken, then the apples.
2. In a small bowl, combine the mustard, honey, salt, and pepper and mix well. Pour the mixture over the ingredients in the slow cooker.
3. Cover and cook on low for 6 hours or on high for 3 hours, or until the chicken is cooked through and the apples and onions are tender. Serve.

Appliance Tip: To cook this recipe on the stovetop, add 2 tablespoons of olive oil. Heat the olive oil in a saucepan and add the onion; cook and stir for 3 minutes. Add the chicken; cook and stir until lightly browned about 5 minutes. Then add the apple and the mustard-honey mixture. Simmer over low heat for 15 to 20 minutes, or until the chicken is cooked through.

Nutrition:
- Calories: 309 Total Fat: 7 g
- Saturated Fat: 2 g Sodium: 369 mg
- Phosphorus: 258 mg Potassium: 465 mg
- Carbohydrates: 30 g Fiber: 4 g
- Protein: 30 g Sugar: 22 g Sugar: 13 g

98. Herbed Chicken and Veggies

Preparation Time: 25 minutes
Cooking Time: 7 hours
Servings: 6
Ingredients:
- 4 large carrots, peeled and sliced
- 1 yellow onion, chopped
- 6 boneless skinless chicken thighs, cut into strips (about 24 ounces)
- 1 teaspoon dried Italian seasoning
- 1/8 teaspoon salt
- 1/8 teaspoon freshly ground black pepper
- 1/3 cup water

Directions:
1. In a 4 to a 5-quart slow cooker, combine the carrots and onion.
2. Sprinkle the chicken with Italian seasoning, salt, and pepper and place on top of the vegetables in the slow cooker. Add the water.
3. Cover and cook on low for 5 to 7 hours. Stir and serve.

Reduce Protein Tip: To make this a medium-protein recipe, use 16 ounces of chicken thighs. The protein content will decrease to 22 g per serving.

Nutrition:
- Calories: 261 Total Fat: 7 g
- Saturated Fat: 2 g
- Sodium: 227 mg
- Phosphorus: 283 mg
- Potassium: 587 mg
- Carbohydrates: 15 g
- Fiber: 3 g Protein: 33 g
- Sugar: 5 g

99. Aussie Turkey
Preparation Time: 25 minutes
Cooking Time: 20 minutes
Servings: 4
Ingredients:
- ¼ cup mayonnaise
- 1 tablespoon onion powder
- 1 tablespoon olive oil
- 1 cup sliced fresh mushrooms
- 2 tablespoons chopped fresh parsley
- 4 skinless, boneless turkey breast halves - pounded to ½-inch thickness
- 1/8 teaspoon black pepper
- ½ cup prepared yellow mustard
- ½ cup honey

Directions:
1. Rub the chicken breasts with the black pepper, cover, and refrigerate for 30 minutes.
2. Preheat oven to 350 degrees F.
3. In a medium bowl, combine the mustard, honey, mayonnaise, and onion powder. Remove half of the sauce, cover, and refrigerate to serve later.
4. Heat oil in a large skillet over medium heat. Place the breasts in the skillet and sauté for 3 to 5 minutes per side, or until browned. Remove from skillet and place the breasts into a 9x13 inch baking dish. Apply the honey mustard sauce to each breast, then layer each breast with mushrooms and bacon.
5. Bake in preheated oven for 15 minutes. Garnish with parsley and serve with the reserved honey mustard sauce.

Nutrition:
- Calories: 388
- Total Fat: 13.8 g
- Saturated Fat: 2.8 g
- Cholesterol: 69 mg
- Sodium: 504 mg
- Total Carbohydrate: 42.2 g
- Dietary Fiber: 1.5 g
- Total Sugar: 36.9 g
- Protein: 27.4 g
- Calcium: 32 mg
- Iron: 2 mg
- Potassium: 149 mg
- Phosphorus: 117 mg

100. Coriander Chicken with Pineapple Salsa
Preparation Time: 30 minutes
Cooking Time: 15 minutes
Servings: 4
Ingredients:
- 1 skinless, boneless chicken breast
- 1 teaspoon black pepper
- 1 tablespoon ground coriander seed
- 2 tablespoons olive oil
- 1 pineapple - peeled, seeded, and chopped
- ⅓ Red onion, chopped
- 1 red Chile pepper, seeded and chopped
- 1 tablespoon chopped fresh cilantro
- ½ teaspoon black pepper

Directions:
1. Sprinkle chicken breast with and 1 teaspoon black pepper; set aside for 10 minutes. Evenly coat with ground coriander.
2. Heat the olive oil in a skillet over medium heat. Cook the chicken breast, browning well on both sides until no longer pink in the center.

Remove from heat, allow the breast to cool before slicing.
3. In a bowl, mix the pineapple, onion, chile pepper, fresh cilantro, and ½ teaspoon black pepper. Pour salsa over sliced chicken breast and serve.

Nutrition:
- Calories: 146
- Total Fat: 8.4 g
- Saturated Fat: 1.4 g
- Cholesterol: 16 mg
- Sodium: 12 mg
- Total Carbohydrate: 12.8 g
- Dietary Fiber: 2.6 g
- Total Sugar: 8.8 g
- Protein: 7.2 g
- Calcium: 37 mg
- Iron: 1 mg
- Potassium: 168 mg
- Phosphorus: 110 mg

101. Honey Chicken Kabobs

Preparation Time: 15 minutes
Cooking Time: 15 minutes
Servings: 4
Ingredients:
- ¼ cup olive oil
- ⅓ cup honey
- ⅓ cup Worcestershire sauce
- ¼ teaspoon ground black pepper
- 8 skinless, boneless chicken breast halves - cut into 1-inch cubes
- 2 cloves garlic
- 5 small onions, cut into 2-inch pieces
- 2 red bell peppers, cut into 2-inch pieces
- Skewers

Directions:
1. In a large bowl, whisk together oil, honey, Worcestershire sauce, and pepper. Before adding chicken, reserve a small amount of marinade for brushing onto kabobs while cooking. Place the chicken, garlic, onions, and peppers in the bowl, and marinate in the refrigerator for at least 2 hours (the longer, the better).
2. Preheat the grill for high heat.
3. Drain marinade from the chicken and vegetables, and discard marinade. Thread chicken and vegetables alternately onto the skewers.
4. Lightly oil the grill grate. Place the skewers on the grill. Cook for 12 to 15 minutes, until chicken juices run clear. Turn and brush with reserved marinade frequently.

Nutrition:
- Calories: 184
- Total Fat: 7 g
- Saturated Fat: 1.6 g
- Cholesterol: 43 mg
- Sodium: 102 mg
- Total Carbohydrate: 13.5 g
- Dietary Fiber: 0.9 g
- Total Sugar: 11.3 g
- Protein: 17.3 g
- Calcium: 10 mg
- Iron: 1 mg
- Potassium: 87 mg
- Phosphorus: 60 mg

102. Chicken Scampi

Preparation Time: 10 minutes
Cooking Time: 20 minutes
Servings: 4
Ingredients:
- ½ cup butter
- ¼ cup olive oil
- 1 teaspoon dried parsley
- 1 teaspoon dried basil
- ¼ teaspoon dried oregano
- 3 cloves garlic, minced
- ¾ teaspoon salt
- 1 tablespoon lemon juice
- 4 boneless chicken breast halves, sliced lengthwise into thirds

Directions:
1. Chop the green onions and red peppers.
2. Trim the ends off the Brussels sprouts and boil or steam until just tender.
3. Cook pasta according to directions on the package but omitting the salt.
4. While macaroni is cooking, drain Brussels sprouts and set aside.
5. Heat butter and oil and sauté green onions in skillet.
6. Add red peppers and Brussels sprouts, stirring until just golden on the edges.
7. Add soy sauce and let vegetable mixture stand covered until macaroni is done.
8. Heat chicken in the microwave if needed.
9. Toss macaroni, chicken, and cooked vegetables in a bowl.
10. Serve immediately while hot.

Nutrition:
- Calories: 402
- Total Fat: 27.6 g
- Saturated Fat: 12 g
- Cholesterol: 138 mg
- Sodium: 480 mg
- Total Carbohydrate: 0.6 g
- Dietary Fiber: 0.1 g
- Total Sugar: 0.1 g
- Protein: 37 g
- Calcium: 26 mg
- Iron: 1 mg
- Potassium: 253 mg
- Phosphorus: 112 mg

103. Chicken with Quinoa and Wild Rice

Preparation Time: 10 minutes
Cooking Time: 40 minutes
Servings: 4
Ingredients:
- ½ cup kale
- 1 cup red onion
- 10 garlic cloves
- 1 tablespoon olive oil
- 6 tablespoons lemon juice
- 1 tablespoon black pepper
- 1 cup quinoa, uncooked
- 1 cup white rice, uncooked
- 4 cups low-sodium chicken broth
- 2 pounds boneless, skinless chicken breast
- 5 tablespoons fresh basil

Directions:
1. Preheat oven to 375°F.
2. Chop kale. Chop the red onion and garlic.
3. Add olive oil, 4 tablespoons of lemon juice, pepper, onion, garlic, quinoa and rice, and chicken broth to a 9-inch x 13-inch baking pan. Mix ingredients together.

4. Add kale on top of the rice mixture.
5. Add chicken breast on top of kale.
6. Cover with foil and bake for 45 minutes or until chicken is done and the majority of chicken broth has been absorbed.
7. Let sit for 5-10 minutes. While the dish is cooling, chop fresh parsley and combine with the remaining 2 tablespoons of lemon juice. Sprinkle on top and enjoy!

Nutrition:
- Calories: 146
- Total Fat: 2.7 g
- Saturated Fat: 0.4 g
- Cholesterol: 11 mg
- Sodium: 40 mg
- Total Carbohydrate: 21.8 g
- Dietary Fiber: 2.4 g
- Total Sugar: 1 g
- Protein. 8.7 g
- Calcium: 27 mg
- Iron: 1 mg
- Potassium: 270 mg
- Phosphorus: 206 mg

104. Pineapple and Mint Lamb Chops

Preparation Time: 10 minutes
Cooking Time: 10 minutes
Servings: 4
Ingredients:
- ½ tablespoon olive oil
- 2 tablespoons pineapple juice
- ¼ tablespoon chopped fresh mint
- Salt and pepper to taste
- 4 lamb chops

Directions:
1. Stir together olive oil, pineapple juice, and mint in a small bowl. Season with salt and pepper to taste. Place lamb chops in a shallow dish, and brush with the olive oil mixture. Marinate in the refrigerator for 1 hour.
2. Preheat grill for high heat.
3. Lightly oil grill grate. Place lamb chops on the grill and discard marinade. Cook for 10 minutes, turning once or to the desired doneness.

Nutrition:
- Calories: 137
- Total Fat: 6.4 g
- Saturated Fat: 1.9 g
- Cholesterol: 57 mg
- Sodium: 49 mg
- Total Carbohydrate: 0.8 g
- Dietary Fiber: 0 g
- Total Sugar: 0.7 g

105. Maple-Brined Pork Loin

Preparation Time: 15 minutes
Cooking Time: 60 minutes
Servings: 4
- 1-quart cold water
- 1/3 cup maple syrup
- 3 cloves garlic, crushed
- 3 tablespoons chopped fresh ginger
- 2 teaspoons dried rosemary
- 1 tablespoon cracked black pepper
- 1 boneless pork loin roast
- Salt and freshly ground black pepper
- 1 tablespoon olive oil
- 2 tablespoons maple syrup
- 2 tablespoons Dijon mustard

Directions:
1. Mix water, salt, 1/3 cup maple syrup, garlic, ginger, rosemary, and black pepper in a large bowl. Place pork loin in brine mixture and refrigerate for 8 to 10 hours.
2. Remove pork from brine, pat dry, and season all sides with salt and black pepper.
3. Preheat oven to 325 degrees F.
4. Heat olive oil in an oven-proof skillet over high heat. Cook pork, turning to brown each side, about 10 minutes' total.
5. Transfer skillet to the oven and roast until pork is browned, about 40 minutes.
6. Mix 2 tablespoons of maple syrup and Dijon mustard together in a small bowl.
7. Remove pork roast from the oven and spread maple syrup mixture on all sides. Cook for an additional 15 minutes, until the pork is no longer pink in the center. An instant-read thermometer inserted into the center should read 145 degrees F.

Nutrition:
- Calories: 158
- Total Fat: 5 g
- Saturated Fat: 0.9 g
- Cholesterol: 16 mg
- Sodium: 106 mg
- Total Carbohydrate: 23.1 g
- Dietary Fiber: 1.5 g
- Total Sugar: 15.9 g

106. Beef Stir-Fry
Preparation Time: 5 minutes
Cooking Time: 15 minutes
Servings: 4
Ingredients:
- 4 cups water
- 2 tablespoons cornstarch
- 2 teaspoons honey
- 6 tablespoons Worcestershire sauce
- 1 tablespoon minced fresh ginger
- 1-pound boneless beef round steak, cut into thin strips
- 1 tablespoon olive oil
- 3 cups broccoli florets
- 2 carrots, thinly sliced
- 1 (6-ounce) package frozen pea pods, thawed
- 2 tablespoons chopped onion
- 1 (8-ounce) can sliced water chestnuts, untrained
- 1 cup cabbage
- ½ cup kale, chopped
- 1 tablespoon olive oil

Directions:
1. Combine corn-starch, honey, and Worcestershire sauce, in a small bowl until smooth. Stir in ginger; toss the beef in the sauce to coat.
2. Heat 1 tablespoon oil in a large skillet over medium-high heat. Cook and stir broccoli, carrots, pea pods, and onion for 1 minute. Stir in water chestnuts, cabbage, and kale; cover and simmer until vegetables are tender, about 4 minutes. Remove from skillet and keep warm.
3. In the same skillet, heat 1 tablespoon of oil over medium-high heat. Cook and stir beef until the desired degree of doneness, about 2 minutes per side

for medium. Return vegetables to skillet; cook and stir until heated through for about 3 minutes.

Nutrition:
- Calories 139
- Total Fat 3.9 g
- Saturated Fat 0.8 g
- Cholesterol 12 mg
- Sodium 972 mg
- Total Carbohydrate 18.7 g
- Dietary Fiber 4 g
- Total Sugar 5.8 g

107. Pork Picadillo
Preparation Time: 25 minutes
Cooking Time: 20 minutes
Servings: 4
Ingredients:
- 2 tablespoons olive oil
- 1 onion, diced
- 2 cloves garlic, crushed
- 2 ½ pounds ground pork
- Salt and pepper to taste
- 1 yellow bell pepper, cut into thin strips
- 1 green bell pepper, cut into thin strips
- 1 red bell pepper, cut into thin strips
- ½ cup kale, chopped

Directions:
1. Heat the olive oil in a large skillet over medium heat. Cook and stir the onion and garlic in the oil until tender, about 5 minutes. Remove the onion and garlic from the pan and set aside.
2. Crumble the pork into the skillet and cook until no longer pink. Return the onion and garlic to the skillet and stir through the pork. Season with salt and pepper. Cover the skillet and cook the mixture for 5 minutes.
3. Stir the green bell pepper, red bell pepper, yellow bell pepper into the mixture; cover and cook for another 5 minutes. Add the kale to the skillet and stir just before serving.

Nutrition:
- Calories: 163
- Total Fat: 9 g
- Saturated Fat: 1.6 g
- Cholesterol: 39 mg
- Sodium: 36 mg
- Total Carbohydrate: 6.2 g
- Dietary Fiber: 1.2 g
- Total Sugar: 2.7 g
- Protein: 14.9 g
- Calcium: 26 mg
- Iron: 1 mg
- Potassium: 367 mg
- Phosphorus: 241 mg

108. Beef Bulgogi
Preparation Time: 10 minutes
Cooking Time: 5 minutes
Servings: 4
Ingredients:
- 1-pound flank steak, thinly sliced
- 5 tablespoons Worcestershire sauce
- 2 ½ tablespoons honey
- ¼ cup chopped green onion
- 2 tablespoons minced garlic
- 2 tablespoons olive oil
- ½ teaspoon ground black pepper

Directions:
1. Place the beef in a shallow dish. Combine Worcestershire sauce, honey, green onion, garlic, olive oil, and ground black pepper in a small bowl. Pour over beef. Cover and

refrigerate for at least 1 hour or overnight.
2. Preheat an outdoor grill for high heat, and lightly oil the grate.
3. Quickly grill beef on the hot grill until slightly charred and cooked through, 1 to 2 minutes per side

Nutrition:
- Calories: 348
- Total Fat: 16.5 g
- Saturated Fat: 4.9 g
- Cholesterol: 62 mg
- Sodium: 272 mg
- Total Carbohydrate: 16.6 g
- Dietary Fiber: 0.4 g
- Total Sugar: 14.7 g

109. Creamy Chicken with Cider
Preparation Time: 25 minutes
Cooking Time: 20 minutes
Servings: 4
Ingredients:
- 4 bone-in chicken breasts
- 2 tbsp. of lightly salted butter
- ¾ cup of apple cider vinegar
- ⅔ cup of rich unsweetened coconut milk or cream
- Kosher pepper

Directions:
1. Melt the butter in a skillet over medium heat.
2. Season the chicken with the pepper and add to the skillet. Cook over low heat for approx. 20 minutes.
3. Remove the chicken from the heat and set aside in a dish.
4. In the same skillet, add the cider and bring to a boil until most of it has evaporated.
5. Add the coconut cream and let cook for 1 minute until slightly thickened.
6. Pour the cider cream over the cooked chicken and serve.

Nutrition:
- Calories: 86.76
- Carbohydrate: 1.88 g
- Protein: 1.5 g
- Sodium: 93.52 mg
- Potassium: 74.65 mg
- Phosphorus: 36.54 mg
- Dietary Fiber: 0.1 g
- Fat: 8.21 g

110. Exotic Palabok
Preparation Time: 25 minutes
Cooking Time: 15 minutes
Servings: 6
Ingredients:
- 12 oz. rice noodles.
- 1 ½ cups of medium shrimp, peeled and deveined
- ⅔ cup of white onion, chopped
- 1 spring onion, sliced
- 3 tbsp. of canola oil
- 1-pound, lean ground turkey
- 2 cups of firm tofu, chopped
- 2 packs of shrimp or ordinary gravy mix
- 5 hard-boiled eggs
- 1 lemon
- ½ cup of pork rinds (optional)

Directions:
1. Boil rice noodles until nice and soft. Keep aside.
2. Boil the peeled shrimp for 2-3 minutes in a pot with plain water.
3. In a wok or shallow pan, sauté the garlic and onion with the oil. Add the ground turkey, tofu, and shrimps.

4. Dissolve the gravy mix in water or as per package instructions.
5. Combine the rice noodles, tofu, onions, and the gravy mix with ½ cup of pork rind (optional).
6. Slice the egg and lemons.
7. Serve with egg and lemons on top.

Nutrition:
- Calories: 305
- Carbohydrate: 39.14 g
- Protein: 17.6 g
- Sodium: 536 mg
- Potassium: 243.52 mg
- Phosphorus: 180.41 mg
- Dietary Fiber: 0.9 g

111. Vegetarian Gobi Curry
Preparation Time: 25 minutes
Cooking Time: 15 minutes
Servings: 4
Ingredients:
- 2 cups of cauliflower florets
- 2 tbsp. of unsalted butter
- 1 medium dry white onion, thinly chopped
- ½ cup of green peas (frozen if wish)
- 1 tsp. of fresh ginger, chopped
- ½ tsp. of turmeric
- 1 tsp of garam masala
- ¼ tsp. cayenne pepper
- 1 tbsp. of water

Directions:
1. Heat a skillet over medium heat with the butter and sauté the onions until caramelized (golden brown).
2. Add the spices, e.g., ginger, garam masala turmeric, and cayenne.
3. Add the cauliflower and the (frozen) peas and stir.

4. Add the water and cover with a lid. Reduce the heat to a low temperature and let cook covered for 10 minutes.
5. Serve with white rice.

Nutrition:
- Calories: 91.04
- Carbohydrate: 7.3 g
- Protein: 2.19 g
- Sodium: 39.38 mg
- Potassium: 209.58 mg
- Phosphorus: 42 mg
- Dietary Fiber: 3 g
- Fat: 6.4 g

112. Marinated Shrimp and Pasta
Preparation Time: 10 minutes
Cooking Time: 20 minutes
Servings: 10
Ingredients:
- 12 oz. of three-colored penne pasta
- ½ pound of cooked shrimp
- ½ red bell pepper, diced
- ½ cup of red onion, chopped
- 3 stalks of celery
- 12 baby carrots, cut into thick slices
- 1 cup of cauliflower, cut into small round pieces
- ¼ cup of honey
- ¼ cup balsamic vinegar
- ½ tsp. of black pepper
- ½ tsp. garlic powder
- 1 tbsp. of French mustard
- ¾ cup of olive oil

Directions:
1. Cook pasta for around 10 minutes (or according to packaged instructions).
2. While pasta is boiling, cut all your veggies and place into a large mixing bowl. Add the cooked shrimp.

3. In a mixing bowl, add the honey, vinegar, black pepper, garlic powder, and mustard. While you whisk, slowly incorporate the oil and stir well.
4. Add in the drained pasta with the veggies and shrimp and gently combine everything. Pour the liquid marinade over the pasta and veggies and toss to coat everything evenly.
5. Refrigerate for 3-5 hours before serving. Serve chilled.

Nutrition:
- Calories: 256
- Carbohydrate: 41 g
- Protein: 6.55 g
- Sodium: 242.04 mg
- Potassium: 131.88 mg
- Phosphorus: 86.03 mg
- Dietary Fiber: 2.28 g
- Fat: 16.88 g

113. Steak and Onion Sandwich
Preparation Time: 25 minutes
Cooking Time: 8 minutes
Servings: 4
Ingredients:
- 4 flank steaks (around 4 oz. each)
- 1 medium red onion, sliced
- 1 tbsp. of lemon juice
- 1 tbsp. of Italian seasoning
- 1 tsp. of black pepper
- 1 tbsp. of vegetable oil
- 4 sandwich/burger buns

Directions:
1. Wrap the steak with lemon juice, Italian seasoning, and pepper to taste. Cut into 4 pieces. Heat the vegetable oil in a medium skillet over medium heat.
2. Cook steaks for around 3 minutes on each side until you get a medium to well-done result. Take off and transfer onto a dish with absorbing paper.
3. In the same skillet, sauté the onions until tender and transparent (around 3 minutes).
4. Cut the sandwich bun into half and place 1 piece of steak in each topped with the onions. Serve or wrap with paper or foil and keep in the fridge for the next day.

Nutrition:
- Calories: 315.26
- Carbohydrate: 8.47 g
- Protein: 38.33 g
- Sodium: 266.24 mg
- Potassium: 238.2 mg
- Phosphorus: 364.25 mg
- Dietary Fiber: 0.76 g
- Fat: 13.22 g

114. Zesty Crab Cakes
Preparation Time: 25 minutes
Cooking Time: 6 minutes
Servings: 6
Ingredients:
- 9 oz. (250 grams) of crab meat
- ⅓ cup of green or red bell pepper, thinly chopped
- ⅓ cup of low salt crackers, crushed
- ¼ cup of low-fat mayonnaise
- 1 tbsp. of dry mustard
- ½ tsp. of pepper
- 2 tbsp. of lemon juice
- ½ tsp. of lemon zest
- 1 tsp. of garlic powder
- 2 tbsp. of vegetable oil

Directions:
1. Mix all the ingredients except for the oil until uniform. Divide into 6 flat patties (around 5 inches in diameter).
2. Heat the vegetable oil in the skillet and shallow fry the patties for 2-3 minutes on each side (or until golden brown).
3. Serve warm on a dish with absorbing paper.

Nutrition:
- Calories: 144.42
- Carbohydrate: 5.12 g
- Protein: 8.47 g
- Sodium: 212.31 mg
- Potassium: 195 mg
- Phosphorus: 127.42 mg
- Dietary Fiber: 1.02 g
- Fat: 9.2 g

115. Tofu Hoisin Sauté

Preparation Time: 15 minutes
Cooking Time: 20 minutes
Servings: 4
Ingredients:
- 2 tablespoons of hoisin sauce
- 2 tablespoons of rice vinegar
- 1 teaspoon of cornstarch
- 2 tablespoons of olive oil
- 1 (15-ounce) package extra-firm tofu, cut into 1-inch cubes
- 2 cups of unpeeled cubed eggplant
- 2 scallions, white and green parts, sliced
- 2 teaspoons of minced garlic
- 1 jalapeño pepper, minced
- 2 tablespoons of chopped fresh cilantro

Directions:
1. In a small bowl, whisk together the hoisin sauce, rice vinegar, and cornstarch and set aside.
2. In a large skillet over medium-high heat, heat the olive oil. Add the tofu, and sauté gently until golden brown, about 10 minutes, and transfer to a plate.
3. Reduce the heat to medium. Add the eggplant, scallions, garlic, jalapeño pepper, and sauté until tender and fragrant, about 6 minutes.
4. Stir in the reserved sauce, and toss until the sauce thickens for about 2 minutes. Stir in the tofu and cilantro, and serve hot.

Low-sodium Tip: Hoisin sauce is made with soy sauce, containing a hefty amount of sodium per serving. This recipe would still be tasty while slightly less intensely flavored if you use 1 tablespoon of hoisin sauce instead of 2 tablespoons.

Nutrition:
- Calories: 105
- Total Fat: 4 g
- Total Fat: 1 g
- Cholesterol: 0 mg
- Sodium: 234 mg
- Carbohydrates: 9 g
- Fiber: 2 g
- Phosphorus: 105 mg
- Potassium: 192 mg
- Protein: 8 g

116. Zucchini Noodles with Spring Vegetables

Preparation Time: 20 minutes
Cooking Time: 10 minutes
Servings: 6
Ingredients:
- 6 zucchinis, cut into long noodles
- 1 cup of halved snow peas
- 1 cup (3-inch pieces) of asparagus
- 1 tablespoon of olive oil
- 1 teaspoon of minced fresh garlic
- 1 tablespoon of freshly squeezed lemon juice
- 2 tablespoons of chopped fresh basil leaves

Directions:
1. Fill a medium saucepan with water, place over medium-high heat, and bring to a boil.
2. Reduce the heat to medium, and blanch the zucchini ribbons, snow peas, and asparagus by submerging them in the water for 1 minute. Drain and rinse immediately under cold water.
3. Pat the vegetables dry with paper towels and transfer to a large bowl.
4. Place a medium skillet over medium heat, and add the olive oil. Add the garlic, and sauté until tender, about 3 minutes.
5. Add the lemon juice
6. Add the zucchini mixture and basil and toss until well combined.
7. Serve immediately.

Nutrition:
- Calories: 52 Total Fat: 2 g
- Total Fat: 0 g Cholesterol: 0 mg
- Sodium: 7 mg
- Carbohydrates: 4 g
- Fiber: 1 g Phosphorus: 40 mg
- Potassium: 197 mg
- Protein: 2 g

117. Stir-Fried Vegetables

Preparation Time: 15 minutes
Cooking Time: 15 minutes
Servings: 4
Ingredients:
- 2 teaspoons of olive oil
- ½ medium red onion, sliced
- 1 tablespoon of grated peeled fresh ginger
- 2 teaspoons of minced garlic
- 2 cups of broccoli florets
- 2 cups of cauliflower florets
- 1 red bell pepper, diced
- 1 cup of sliced carrots

Directions:
1. In a large skillet over medium-high heat, heat the olive oil.
2. Add the onion, ginger, and garlic and sauté until softened, about 3 minutes.
3. Add the broccoli, cauliflower, bell pepper, carrots, and sauté until tender, about 10 minutes.
4. Serve hot.

Nutrition:
- Calories: 50
- Total Fat: 1 g
- Total Fat: 0 g
- Cholesterol: 0 mg
- Sodium: 26 mg
- Carbohydrates: 6 g
- Fiber: 2 g
- Phosphorus: 36 mg
- Potassium: 198 mg
- Protein: 1 g

118. Lime Asparagus Spaghetti

Preparation Time: 5 minutes
Cooking Time: 20 minutes
Servings: 6
Ingredients:
- 1 pound of asparagus spears, trimmed and cut into 2-inch pieces
- 2 teaspoons of olive oil
- 2 teaspoons of minced garlic
- 2 teaspoons of all-purpose flour
- 1 cup of homemade rice milk (here, or use unsweetened store-bought) or almond milk
- Juice and zest of ½ lemon
- 1 tablespoon of chopped fresh thyme
- Freshly ground black pepper
- 2 cups of cooked spaghetti
- ¼ cup of grated Parmesan cheese

Directions:
1. Fill a large saucepan with water and bring to a boil over high heat. Add the asparagus and blanch until crisp-tender, about 2 minutes. Drain and set aside.
2. In a large skillet over medium-high heat, heat the olive oil. Add the garlic, and sauté until softened, about 2 minutes. Whisk in the flour to create a paste, about 1 minute. Whisk in the rice milk, lemon juice, lemon zest, and thyme.
3. Reduce the heat to medium and cook the sauce, constantly whisking until thickened and creamy, about 3 minutes.
4. Season the sauce with pepper.
5. Stir in the spaghetti and the asparagus.
6. Serve the pasta topped with the Parmesan cheese.

Nutrition:
- Calories: 127
- Total Fat: 3 g
- Total Fat: 1 g
- Cholesterol: 4 mg
- Sodium: 67 mg
- Carbohydrates: 19 g
- Fiber: 2 g
- Phosphorus 109 mg
- Potassium: 200 mg
- Protein: 6 g

119. Garden Crustless Quiche

Preparation Time: 25 minutes
Cooking Time: 20 minutes
Servings: 6
Ingredients:
- 6 eggs
- 2 egg whites
- ¼ cup of homemade rice milk (here or use unsweetened store-bought)
- ¼ cup of shredded Swiss cheese, divided
- ¼ teaspoon of freshly ground black pepper
- 1 teaspoon of unsalted butter, plus more for the pie plate
- 1 teaspoon of minced garlic
- 1 scallion, white and green parts, chopped
- 1 yellow zucchini, chopped
- ½ cup of shredded stemmed kale

Directions:
1. In a medium bowl, beat the eggs, egg whites, rice milk, half the Swiss cheese, and the pepper until well blended, and set aside.
2. Preheat the oven to 350°F.
3. Grease a 9-inch pie plate with butter and set aside.

4. In a medium skillet over medium-high heat, melt 1 teaspoon of butter. Add the garlic and scallion, and sauté until softened, about 2 minutes.
5. Add the zucchini and kale, and sauté until wilted, about 3 minutes.
6. Transfer the vegetables from the skillet to the pie plate and spread the vegetables evenly across the bottom.
7. Pour the egg mixture into the pie plate, and sprinkle with the remaining half of the Swiss cheese.
8. Bake until the quiche is puffed and lightly browned, 15 to 20 minutes.
9. Serve hot, warm, or cold.

Ingredient Tip: Yellow zucchini, sometimes called summer squash, is usually lined up in a bin next to the more common green variety. You can interchange green with yellow in this dish.

Nutrition:
- Calories: 120
- Total Fat: 8 g
- Total Fat: 4 g
- Cholesterol: 221 mg
- Sodium: 93 mg
- Carbohydrates: 3 g
- Fiber: 0 g
- Phosphorus 120 mg
- Potassium: 189 mg
- Protein: 9 g

120. Lentil Veggie Burgers

Preparation Time: 15 minutes
Cooking Time: 10 minutes
Servings: 4
Ingredients:
- 2½ cups cooked white rice
- ½ cup cooked red lentils, drained and rinsed
- 2 eggs, lightly beaten
- 2 tablespoons chopped fresh parsley
- 2 teaspoons chopped fresh basil leaves
- Juice and zest of 1 lime
- 1 teaspoon minced garlic
- 1 tablespoon olive oil

Directions:
1. In a food processor (or blender), pulse the rice, lentils, eggs, parsley, basil, lime juice, lime zest, and garlic until the mixture holds together.
2. Transfer the rice mixture to a medium bowl, and set in the refrigerator until it firms up for about 1 hour.
3. Form the rice mixture into 4 patties.
4. In a large skillet over medium-high heat, heat the olive oil.
5. Add the veggie patties and cook until golden, about 5 minutes. Flip the patties over. Cook the other side for 5 minutes.
6. Transfer the burgers to a paper towel–lined plate.
7. Serve the veggie burgers hot with your favorite toppings.

Nutrition:
- Calories: 247
- Total Fat: 7 g
- Total Fat: 2 g
- Cholesterol: 106 mg
- Sodium: 36 mg
- Carbohydrates: 31 g
- Fiber: 3 g
- Phosphorus 120 mg
- Potassium: 183 mg
- Protein: 8 g

121. Baked Cauliflower Rice Cakes

Preparation Time: 20 minutes
Cooking Time: 10 minutes
Servings: 6
Ingredients:
- Olive oil for the pan
- 2 cups of chopped blanched cauliflower (see Cooking tip)
- 2 cups of cooked white basmati rice
- ¼ cup of plain yogurt
- 2 eggs, lightly beaten
- ½ cup of grated Cheddar cheese
- ¼ teaspoon of ground nutmeg
- Freshly ground black pepper

Directions:
1. Preheat the oven to 350°F.
2. Lightly coat 6 cups of a standard muffin tin with olive oil.
3. In a large bowl, mix the cauliflower, rice, yogurt, eggs, cheese, and nutmeg.
4. Season the mixture with pepper.
5. Evenly divide the cauliflower mixture among the 6 prepared muffin cups.
6. Bake until golden and slightly puffy for about 20 minutes.
7. Let them stand for 5 minutes, then run a knife around the edges to loosen.
8. Serve hot, warm, or cold.

Nutrition:
- Calories: 141
- Total Fat: 5 g
- Total Fat: 3 g
- Cholesterol: 82 mg
- Sodium: 98 mg
- Carbohydrates: 18 g
- Fiber: 1 g
- Phosphorus 119 mg
- Potassium: 178 mg
- Protein: 7 g

122. Marinated Paprika Chicken

Preparation Time: 25 minutes
Cooking Time: 3 hours
Servings: 4
Ingredients:
- ½ cup chopped onion, sweet
- ¼ cup oil, olive
- 2 tbsp. lemon juice, freshly squeezed if available
- 1 tbsp. chopped oregano, fresh
- 1 tsp. minced garlic
- 1 tsp. paprika, smoked
- 4 x 3-oz. chicken thighs, skinless, boneless

Directions:
1. Add lemon juice, oil, onion, paprika, oregano, and garlic to the food processor. Puree.
2. Next, pour the mixture into a large zipper-top plastic bag. Add chicken.
3. Press air from bag and seal. Place in refrigerator, then allow to marinate for about two hours. Turn the bag a few times while marinating.
4. Preheat oven to 400F. Place chicken thighs in a baking dish. Discard leftover marinade.
5. Roast chicken till cooked fully through, 30-35 minutes. Serve while hot.

Nutrition:
For each serving (1 chicken thigh)
- Calories: 196 Fat: 11 g
- Cholesterol: 47 mg
- Carbs: 3 g Sugar: 2 g
- Fiber: 2 g Protein: 18 g
- Sodium: 60 mg Calcium: 17 mg
- Phosphorus: 166 mg
- Potassium: 232 mg

123. Cool Cucumber Salad

Preparation Time: 25 minutes
Cooking Time: 10 minutes
Servings: 6
Ingredients:
- 2 cups of ¼"-thick sliced cucumbers, fresh, peeled, or unpeeled
- 2 tbsp. of salad dressing, Caesar or Italian, no sodium
- Pepper, ground, as desired

Directions:
1. In a medium bowl with a secure lid, combine sliced cucumbers with salad dressing.
2. Cover the bowl with the lid, then shake, coating cucumbers.
3. Sprinkle using pepper. Place in refrigerator. Serve chilled.

Nutrition:
- Calories: 26
- Fat: 1.5 g
- Cholesterol: 0 mg
- Sodium: 73 mg
- Carbs: 2 g
- Protein: 0 g
- Phosphorus: 12 mg
- Potassium: 88 mg
- Fiber: 0 g
- Calcium: 11 mg

124. Sautéed Butternut Squash

Preparation Time: 25 minutes
Cooking Time: 10 minutes
Servings: 8
Ingredients:
- 1 tbsp. of oil, olive
- 4 cups of peeled, de-seeded, cubed squash, butternut
- ½ chopped onion, sweet
- 1 tsp. of chopped thyme, fresh
- A pinch pepper, ground

Directions:
1. Heat oil in a large-sized skillet on med-high heat.
2. Add squash. Sauté till tender, 15-17 minutes.
3. Add thyme and onion. Sauté for five minutes more.
4. Season using ground pepper. Serve while hot.

Nutrition:
For each serving (1 serving)
- Calories: 50
- Fat: 1.5 g
- Cholesterol: 0 mg
- Carbs: 8 g
- Sugar: 2 g
- Fiber: 2 g
- Protein: 2 g
- Sodium: 3 mg
- Calcium: 36 mg
- Phosphorus: 20 mg
- Potassium: 243 mg

125. Herb Roasted Chicken

Preparation Time: 25 minutes
Cooking Time: 20 minutes
Servings: 4
Ingredients:
- 1 lb. of chicken breasts, skinless, boneless
- 1 onion, medium
- 1 or 2 cloves of garlic, fresh
- 2 tbsp. of herb & garlic seasoning
- 1 tsp. of pepper, ground
- ¼ cup of oil, olive

Directions:
1. Chop the garlic and onion. Place in a bowl. Add oil, seasoning, and pepper.
2. Add chicken to marinade and cover. Then, place in the refrigerator for four hours or overnight.
3. Preheat oven to 375F.
4. Cover the cookie sheet with aluminum foil. Place marinated chicken on the foil.
5. Pour the remainder of the marinade over the chicken. Bake in 375F oven for 18-20 minutes.
6. Broil for five extra minutes to brown, if desired. Serve.

Nutrition:
For each serving (4 ounces)
- Calories: 268
- Fat: 16 g
- Cholesterol: 82 mg
- Sodium: 52 mg
- Carbs: 2 g
- Protein: 25 g
- Phosphorus: 250 mg
- Potassium: 489 mg
- Fiber: 0.5 g
- Calcium: 16 mg

126. Seared Scallops
Preparation Time: 25 minutes
Cooking Time: 20 minutes
Servings: 4
Ingredients:
- 1 tbsp. of oil, olive
- 12 oz. of rinsed, patted dry sea scallops
- Pepper, ground, as desired
- 2 tbsp. of lemon juice, freshly squeezed if available
- 1 tsp. each of fresh chopped parsley, thyme, and chives

Directions:
1. Heat oil in a large-sized skillet on med-high.
2. Season scallops lightly using pepper. Add to skillet.
3. Sea scallops and turn once till just cooked fully through and lightly browned for about three to four minutes.
4. Add and stir in lemon juice, chives, parsley, and thyme.
5. Turn scallops, coating in herb sauce. Serve while hot.

Nutrition:
For each serving (3 scallops)
- Calories: 119
- Fat: 4 g
- Cholesterol: 26 mg
- Carbs: 2 g
- Sugar: 0 g
- Fiber: 4 g
- Protein: 12 g
- Sodium: 288 mg
- Calcium: 7 mg
- Phosphorus: 245 mg
- Potassium: 199 mg

127. Dolmas Wrap
Preparation Time: 10 minutes
Cooking Time: 10 minutes
Servings: 2
Ingredients:
- 2 whole wheat wrap
- 6 dolmas (stuffed grape leaves)
- 1 tomato, chopped
- 1 cucumber, chopped
- 2 oz. Greek yogurt
- ½ teaspoon minced garlic

- ¼ cup lettuce, chopped
- 2 oz. Feta, crumbled

Directions:
1. The mixing bowl combines chopped tomato, cucumber, Greek yogurt, minced garlic, lettuce, and Feta.
2. When the mixture is homogenous, transfer it to the center of every wheat wrap.
3. Arrange dolma over the vegetable mixture.
4. Carefully wrap the wheat wraps.

Nutrition:
- Calories: 341 Fat: 12.9 g
- Fiber: 9.2 g
- Carbs: 52.4 g
- Protein: 13.2 g

128. Salad al Tonno
Preparation Time: 15 minutes
Cooking Time: 15 minutes
Servings: 2
Ingredients:
- 1 ½ cup lettuce leaves, teared
- ½ teaspoon garlic powder
- ½ teaspoon salt
- ½ teaspoon ground black pepper
- 1 tablespoon lemon juice
- 1 teaspoon olive oil

Directions:
1. Add lettuce leaves, salt, garlic powder, ground black pepper. Lemon juice, and olive oil.
2. Give a good shake to the salad.
3. Salad can be stored in the fridge for up to 3 hours.

Nutrition:
- Calories: 235
- Fat: 12 g
- Fiber: 1 g Carbs: 6.5 g
- Protein: 23.4 g

129. Arlecchino Rice Salad
Preparation Time: 10 minutes
Cooking Time: 15 minutes
Servings: 3
Ingredients:
- ½ cup white rice, dried
- 1 cup chicken stock
- 1 zucchini, shredded
- 2 tablespoons capers
- 1 carrot, shredded
- 1 tomato, chopped
- 1 tablespoon apple cider vinegar
- ½ teaspoon salt
- 2 tablespoons fresh parsley, chopped
- 1 tablespoon canola oil

Directions:
1. Put rice in the pan.
2. Add chicken stock and boil it with the closed lid for 15-20 minutes or until rice absorbs all water.
3. Meanwhile, in the mixing bowl, combine shredded zucchini, capers, carrot, and tomato.
4. Add fresh parsley.
5. Make the dressing: mix up together canola oil, salt, and apple cider vinegar.
6. Chill the cooked rice a little and add it in the salad bowl to the vegetables.
7. Add dressing and mix up salad well.

Nutrition:
- Calories: 183 Fat: 5.3 g
- Fiber: 2.1 g Carbs: 30.4 g
- Protein: 3.8 g

130. Greek Salad

Preparation Time: 10 minutes
Cooking Time: 0 minutes
Servings: 2
Ingredients:
- 2 cups lettuce leaves
- 2 cucumbers
- 1 tablespoon lemon juice
- 1 teaspoon olive oil
- ¼ teaspoon dried oregano
- ½ teaspoon salt
- ¼ teaspoon chili flakes
- 4 oz. Feta cheese

Directions:
1. Chop Feta cheese into small cubes.
2. Chop the lettuce leaves roughly put them in the salad bowl.
3. Then chop cucumbers into the cubes. Add them to the lettuce bowl.
4. For the dressing: whisk together chili flakes, salt, dried oregano, olive oil, and lemon juice.
5. Pour the dressing over the lettuce mixture and mix up well.
6. Sprinkle the salad with Feta cubes and shake gently.

Nutrition:
- Calories: 312
- Fat: 21.2 g
- Fiber: 5.3 g
- Carbs: 23.5 g
- Protein: 11.9 g

131. Baked Vegetables Soup

Preparation Time: 15 minutes
Cooking Time: 5 hours
Servings: 2
Ingredients:
- 1 carrot, peeled
- 1 onion, peeled
- 1 eggplant, peeled
- 2 oz. asparagus, peeled
- 2 tablespoons sour cream
- 1 teaspoon salt
- ½ teaspoon ground black pepper
- 1 tablespoon dried dill
- 2 cups of water

Directions:
1. Place all vegetables in the tray and bake them for 30 minutes at 360F.
2. When the vegetables are tender, chop them roughly and put them in the pan.
3. Add water, dried dill, ground black pepper, salt, and close the lid.
4. Simmer the soup for 10 minutes.
5. After this, gently blend the soup. It should have a soft but not smooth texture.
6. Simmer the soup for 2-3 minutes and remove from the heat.
7. Add more salt if needed.

Nutrition:
- Calories: 128
- Fat: 3.1 g
- Fiber: 11 g
- Carbs: 24.4 g
- Protein: 4.5 g

132. Pesto Chicken Salad

Preparation Time: 15 minutes
Cooking Time: 15 minutes
Servings: 4
Ingredients:
- 1-pound chicken breast, skinless, boneless
- 1 teaspoon salt
- 1 teaspoon ground black pepper
- 1 teaspoon olive oil
- 2 cucumbers, chopped

- 1 cup lettuce, chopped
- 1 red onion, sliced
- 3 tablespoons fresh basil
- 2 oz. Parmesan, grated
- 1 tablespoon walnut
- ½ teaspoon minced garlic
- 1 tablespoon canola oil
- 1 tablespoon lemon juice

Directions:
1. Preheat the grill to 360F.
2. Rub the chicken breast with salt, ground black pepper, and olive oil.
3. Grill the chicken for 7 minutes from each side. The cooked chicken breast should have a crunchy crust.
4. Meanwhile, mix up cucumbers, lettuce, red onion, and mix up the mixture well. Add lemon juice and canola oil. Mix up the salad well again.
5. Make pesto sauce: blend in the blender minced garlic, walnuts, Parmesan, and basil.
6. Chop the cooked grilled chicken breast roughly and put it over the salad.
7. Drizzle the salad with pesto sauce.

Nutrition:
- Calories: 293
- Fat: 13.9 g
- Fiber: 2.9 g
- Carbs: 12.3 g
- Protein: 31.1 g

133. Falafel

Preparation Time: 10 minutes
Cooking Time: 6 minutes
Servings: 4
Ingredients:
- 1 cup chickpeas, soaked, cooked
- 1/3 cup white onion, diced
- 3 garlic cloves, chopped
- 3 tablespoons fresh parsley, chopped
- 1 tablespoon chickpea flour
- ½ teaspoon salt
- ½ teaspoon ground cumin
- ¾ teaspoon ground coriander
- ½ teaspoon chili flakes
- ½ teaspoon cayenne pepper
- ½ teaspoon ground cardamom
- 3 tablespoons olive oil

Directions:
1. Blend chickpeas, onion, garlic cloves, parsley, chickpea flour, salt, ground cumin, ground coriander, chili flakes, and cayenne pepper ground cardamom.
2. When the chickpea mixture is homogenous and smooth, transfer it to the mixing bowl.
3. Make the medium balls from the chickpea mixture.
4. Pour olive oil into the skillet and heat it.
5. Fry the chickpea balls for 2 minutes from each side over medium heat.
6. The cooked falafel should have a light brown color.
7. Dry the falafel with a paper towel if needed.

Nutrition:
- Calories: 283
- Fat: 13.7 g
- Fiber: 9.2 g
- Carbs: 32.6 g
- Protein: 10.1 g

134. Israeli Pasta Salad

Preparation Time: 10 minutes
Cooking Time: 15 minutes
Servings: 2
Ingredients:
- 2 bell peppers, chopped
- 3 oz. Feta cheese, chopped
- 1 red onion, chopped
- 1 tomato, chopped
- 1 cucumber, chopped
- ½ cup elbow macaroni, dried
- 1 teaspoon dried oregano
- 1 tablespoon lemon juice
- 1 teaspoon olive oil
- 1 cup water for macaroni

Directions:
1. Pour water in the pan, add macaroni and boil them according to the
2. Directions of the manufacturer (approx. 15 minutes).
3. Then drain water and chill the macaroni a little.
4. Meanwhile, in the salad bowl, mix up together Feta cheese, bell peppers, onion, tomato, and cucumber.
5. Make the dressing for the salad: combine dried oregano, lemon juice, and olive oil.
6. Add cooked macaroni to the salad bowl and mix up well.
7. Drizzle the salad with dressing and shake gently.

Nutrition:
- Calories: 328
- Fat: 14.8 g
- Fiber: 5.6 g
- Carbs: 40.3 g
- Protein: 12.2 g

135. Artichoke Matzo Mina

Preparation Time: 10 minutes
Cooking Time: 45 minutes
Servings: 6
Ingredients:
- 4 sheets matzo
- ½ cup artichoke hearts
- 1 cup cream cheese
- ½ teaspoon salt
- 1 teaspoon ground black pepper
- 3 tablespoons fresh dill, chopped
- 3 eggs, beaten
- 1 teaspoon canola oil
- ½ cup cottage cheese

Directions:
1. In the bowl combine, salt, ground black pepper, dill, and cottage cheese.
2. Pour canola oil in the skillet, add artichoke hearts and roast them for 2-3 minutes over medium heat. Stir them from time to time.
3. Then add roasted artichoke hearts to the cheese mixture.
4. Add eggs and stir until homogenous. Place one sheet of matzo in the casserole mold.
5. Then spread it with cheese mixture generously.
6. Cover the cheese layer with the second sheet of matzo.
7. Repeat the steps till you use all ingredients.
8. Then preheat oven to 360F.
9. Bake matzo mina for 40 minutes.
10. Cut the cooked meal into the.

Nutrition:
- Calories: 272 Fat: 17.3 g
- Fiber: 4.3 g Carbs: 20.2 g
- Protein: 11.8 g

136. Sautéed Chickpea and Lentil Mix

Preparation Time: 10 minutes
Cooking Time: 50 minutes
Servings: 4
Ingredients:

- 1 cup chickpeas, half-cooked
- 1 cup lentils
- 5 cups chicken stock
- ½ cup fresh cilantro, chopped
- 1 teaspoon salt
- ½ teaspoon chili flakes
- ¼ cup onion, diced
- 1 tablespoon tomato paste

Directions:

1. Place chickpeas in the pan.
2. Add water, salt, and chili flakes.
3. Boil the chickpeas for 30 minutes over medium heat.
4. Then add diced onion, lentils, and tomato paste. Stir well.
5. Close the lid and cook the mix for 15 minutes.
6. After this, add chopped cilantro, stir the meal well and cook it for 5 minutes more.
7. Let the cooked lunch chill a little before serving.

Nutrition:

- Calories: 370
- Fat: 4.3 g
- Fiber: 23.7 g
- Carbs: 61.6 g
- Protein: 23.2 g

137. Buffalo Chicken Lettuce Wraps

Preparation Time: 35 minutes
Cooking Time: 10 minutes
Servings: 2
Ingredients:

- 3 chicken breasts, boneless and cubed
- 20 slices of almond butter lettuce leaves
- ¾ cup cherry tomatoes halved
- 1 avocado, chopped
- ¼ cup green onions, diced
- ½ cup ranch dressing
- ¾ cup hot sauce

Directions:

1. Take a mixing bowl and add chicken cubes and hot sauce, mix. Place in the fridge and let it marinate for 30 minutes.
2. Preheat your oven to 400 degrees F.
3. Place coated chicken on a cookie pan and bake for 9 minutes.
4. Assemble lettuce serving cups with equal amounts of lettuce, green onions, tomatoes, ranch dressing, and cubed chicken. Serve and enjoy!

Nutrition:

- Calories: 106
- Fat: 6g
- Carbohydrates: 2g
- Protein: 5g

138. Crazy Japanese Potato and Beef Croquettes

Preparation Time: 10 minutes
Cooking Time: 20 minutes
Servings: 10
Ingredients:
- 3 medium russet potatoes, peeled and chopped
- 1 tablespoon almond butter
- 1 tablespoon vegetable oil
- 3 onions, diced
- ¾ pound ground beef
- 4 teaspoons light coconut aminos
- All-purpose flour for coating
- 2 eggs, beaten
- Panko bread crumbs for coating
- ½ cup oil, frying

Directions:
1. Take a saucepan and place it over medium-high heat; add potatoes and sunflower seeds water, boil for 16 minutes.
2. Remove water and put potatoes in another bowl, add almond butter and mash the potatoes.
3. Take a frying pan and place it over medium heat, add 1 tablespoon oil and let it heat up.
4. Add onions and stir fry until tender.
5. Add coconut aminos to beef to onions.
6. Keep frying until beef is browned.
7. Mix the beef with the potatoes evenly.
8. Take another frying pan and place it over medium heat; add half a cup of oil.
9. Form croquettes using the mashed potato mixture and coat them with flour, then eggs and finally breadcrumbs. Fry patties until golden on all sides. Enjoy!

Nutrition:
- Calories 239
- Fat 4g
- Carbohydrates 20g
- Protein 10g

139. Spicy Chili Crackers

Preparation Time: 15 minutes
Cooking Time: 60 minutes
Servings: 30 crackers
Ingredients:
- ¾ cup almond flour
- ¼ cup coconut flour
- ½ teaspoon paprika
- ½ teaspoon cumin
- 1 ½ teaspoons chili pepper spice
- 1 teaspoon onion powder
- ½ teaspoon sunflower seeds
- 1 whole egg
- ¼ cup unsalted almond butter

Directions:
1. Preheat your oven to 350 degrees F.
2. Line a baking sheet with parchment paper and keep it on the side.
3. Add ingredients to your food processor and pulse until you have a nice dough.
4. Divide dough into two equal parts.
5. Place one ball on a sheet of parchment paper and cover with another sheet; roll it out.
6. Cut into crackers and repeat with the other ball.
7. Transfer the prepped dough to a baking tray and bake for 8-10 minutes.
8. Remove from oven and serve. Enjoy!

Nutrition:
- Carbs: 2.8g Fiber: 1g
- Protein: 1.6g
- Fat: 4.1g

140. Golden Eggplant Fries

Preparation Time: 10 minutes
Cooking Time: 15 minutes
Servings: 8
Ingredients:
- 2 eggs
- 2 cups almond flour
- 2 tablespoons coconut oil, spray
- 2 eggplant, peeled and cut thinly
- Sunflower seeds and pepper

Directions:
1. Preheat your oven to 400 degrees F.
2. Take a bowl and mix with sunflower seeds and black pepper.
3. Take another bowl and beat eggs until frothy.
4. Dip the eggplant pieces into the eggs.
5. Then coat them with the flour mixture.
6. Add another layer of flour and egg.
7. Then, take a baking sheet and grease with coconut oil on top.
8. Bake for about 15 minutes.

Serve and enjoy!
Nutrition:
- Calories: 212
- Fat: 15.8g
- Carbohydrates: 12.1g
- Protein: 8.6g

141. Traditional Black Bean Chili

Preparation Time: 10 minutes
Cooking Time: 4 hours
Servings: 4
Ingredients:
- 1 ½ cups red bell pepper, chopped
- 1 cup yellow onion, chopped
- 1 ½ cups mushrooms, sliced
- 1 tablespoon olive oil
- 1 tablespoon chili powder
- 2 garlic cloves, minced
- 1 teaspoon chipotle chili pepper, chopped
- ½ teaspoon cumin, ground
- 16 ounces canned black beans, drained and rinsed
- 2 tablespoons cilantro, chopped
- 1 cup tomatoes, chopped

Directions:
1. Add red bell peppers, onion, dill, mushrooms, chili powder, garlic, chili pepper, cumin, black beans, and tomatoes to your Slow Cooker.
2. Stir well. Place lid and cook on high heat for 4 hours. Sprinkle cilantro on top.

Serve and enjoy!
Nutrition:
- Calories: 211
- Fat: 3g
- Carbohydrates: 22g
- Protein: 5g

142. Very Wild Mushroom Pilaf

Preparation Time: 10 minutes
Cooking Time: 3 hours
Servings: 4
Ingredients:
- 1 cup wild rice
- 2 garlic cloves, minced
- 6 green onions, chopped
- 2 tablespoons olive oil
- ½ pound baby Bella mushrooms
- 2 cups water

Directions:
1. Add rice, garlic, onion, oil, mushrooms and water to your Slow Cooker.
2. Stir well until mixed.

3. Place lid and cook on low heat for 3 hours.
4. Stir pilaf and divide between serving platters.

Enjoy!

Nutrition:
- Calories: 210
- Fat: 7g
- Carbohydrates: 16g
- Protein: 4g

143. Green Palak Paneer

Preparation Time: 5 minutes
Cooking Time: 10 minutes
Servings: 4
Ingredients:
- 1-pound spinach
- 2 cups cubed paneer (vegan)
- 2 tablespoons coconut oil
- 1 teaspoon cumin
- 1 chopped up onion
- 1-2 teaspoons hot green chili minced up
- 1 teaspoon minced garlic
- 15 cashews
- 4 tablespoons almond milk
- 1 teaspoon Garam masala
- Flavored vinegar as needed

Directions:
1. Add cashews and milk to a blender and blend well.
2. Set your pot to Sauté mode and add coconut oil; allow the oil to heat up.
3. Add cumin seeds, garlic, green chilies, ginger and sauté for 1 minute.
4. Add onion and sauté for 2 minutes.
5. Add chopped spinach, flavored vinegar and a cup of water.
6. Lock up the lid and cook on HIGH pressure for 10 minutes.
7. Quick-release the pressure
8. Add ½ cup of water and blend to a paste.
9. Add cashew paste, paneer and Garam Masala and stir thoroughly.

Serve over hot rice!

Nutrition:
- Calories 367
- Fat 26g
- Carbohydrates 21g
- Protein 16g

CHAPTER 5:

Fish and Seafood

144. Shrimp Paella

Preparation Time: 5 minutes
Cooking Time: 10 minutes
Servings: 2
Ingredients:
- 1 cup cooked rice
- 1 chopped red onion
- 1 teaspoon paprika
- 1 chopped garlic clove
- 1 tablespoon olive oil
- 6 oz. frozen cooked shrimp
- 1 deseeded and sliced chili pepper
- 1 tablespoon oregano

Directions:
1. Heat the olive oil in a large pan on medium-high heat.
2. Add the onion and garlic and sauté for 2-3 minutes until soft.
3. Now add the shrimp and sauté for a further 5 minutes or until hot.
4. Now add the herbs, spices, chili, and rice with ½ cup boiling water.
5. Stir until everything is warm and the water has been absorbed.
6. Plate up and serve.

Nutrition:
- Calories: 221 Protein: 17 g
- Carbohydrates: 31 g
- Fat: 8 g
- Sodium (Na): 235 mg
- Potassium: (K) 176 mg
- Phosphorus: 189 mg

145. Salmon and Pesto Salad

Preparation Time: 5 minutes
Cooking Time: 15 minutes
Servings: 2
Ingredients:
For the pesto:
- 1 minced garlic clove
- ½ cup fresh arugula
- ¼ cup extra virgin olive oil
- ½ cup fresh basil
- 1 teaspoon black pepper

For the salmon:
- 4 oz. skinless salmon fillet
- 1 tablespoon coconut oil

For the salad:
- ½ juiced lemon
- 2 sliced radishes
- ½ cup iceberg lettuce
- 1 teaspoon black pepper

Directions:
1. Prepare the pesto by blending all the pesto ingredients in a food processor or grinding with a pestle and mortar. Set aside.
2. Add a skillet to the stove on medium-high heat and melt the coconut oil.
3. Add the salmon to the pan.
4. Cook for 7-8 minutes and turn over.
5. Cook for a further 3-4 minutes or until cooked through.

6. Remove fillets from the skillet and allow to rest.
7. Mix the lettuce and the radishes and squeeze over the juice of ½ lemon.
8. Flake the salmon with a fork and mix through the salad.
9. Toss to coat and sprinkle with a little black pepper to serve.

Nutrition:
- Calories: 221 Protein: 13 g
- Carbohydrates: 1 g Fat: 34 g
- Sodium (Na): 80 mg
- Potassium (K): 119 mg
- Phosphorus: 158 mg

146. Baked Fennel and Garlic Sea Bass

Preparation Time: 5 minutes
Cooking Time: 15 minutes
Servings: 2
Ingredients:
- 1 lemon - ½ sliced fennel bulb
- 6 oz. sea bass fillets
- 1 teaspoon black pepper
- 2 garlic cloves

Directions:
1. Preheat the oven to 375°F/Gas Mark 5.
2. Sprinkle black pepper over the sea bass.
3. Slice the fennel bulb and garlic cloves.
4. Add 1 salmon fillet and half the fennel and garlic to one sheet of baking paper or tin foil.
5. Squeeze in ½ lemon juices.
6. Repeat for the other fillet.
7. Fold and add to the oven for 12-15 minutes or until fish is thoroughly cooked through.

8. Meanwhile, add boiling water to your couscous, cover, and allow to steam. Serve with your choice of rice or salad.

Nutrition:
- Calories: 221 Protein: 14 g
- Carbohydrates: 3 g Fat: 2 g
- Sodium (Na): 119 mg
- Potassium (K): 398 mg
- Phosphorus: 149 mg

147. Lemon, Garlic & Cilantro Tuna and Rice

Preparation Time: 5 minutes
Cooking Time: 0 minutes
Servings: 2
Ingredients:
- ½ cup arugula
- 1 tablespoon extra-virgin olive oil
- 1 cup cooked rice
- 1 teaspoon black pepper
- ¼ finely diced red onion
- 1 juiced lemon
- 2 tablespoons chopped fresh cilantro - 1 tuna

Directions:
1. Mix the olive oil, pepper, cilantro, and red onion in a bowl.
2. Stir in the tuna and serve immediately.
3. When ready to eat, serve up with the cooked rice and arugula!

Nutrition:
- Calories: 221 Protein: 11 g
- Carbohydrates: 26 g Fat: 7 g
- Sodium (Na): 143 mg
- Potassium: (K)197 mg
- Phosphorus: 182 mg

148. Cod & Green Bean Risotto

Preparation Time: 4 minutes
Cooking Time: 40 minutes
Servings: 2
Ingredients:
- ½ cup arugula
- 1 finely diced white onion
- 4 oz. cod fillet
- 1 cup white rice
- 2 lemon wedges
- 1 cup boiling water
- ¼ teaspoon black pepper
- 1 cup low sodium chicken broth
- 1 tablespoon extra-virgin olive oil
- ½ cup green beans

Directions:
1. Heat the oil in a large pan on medium heat.
2. Sauté the chopped onion for 5 minutes until soft before adding in the rice and stirring for 1-2 minutes.
3. Combine the broth with boiling water.
4. Add half of the liquid to the pan and stir slowly.
5. Slowly add the rest of the liquid while continuously stirring for up to 20-30 minutes.
6. Stir in the green beans to the risotto.
7. Place the fish on top of the rice, cover, and steam for 10 minutes.
8. Ensure the water does not dry out and keep topping up until the rice is cooked thoroughly.
9. Use your fork to break up the fish fillets and stir into the rice.
10. Sprinkle with freshly ground pepper and a squeeze of fresh lemon to serve.
11. Garnish with the lemon wedges and serve with the arugula.

Nutrition:
- Calories: 221
- Protein: 12 g
- Carbohydrates: 29 g
- Fat: 8 g
- Sodium (Na): 398 mg
- Potassium (K): 347 mg
- Phosphorus: 241 mg

149. Mixed Pepper Stuffed River Trout

Preparation Time: 5 minutes
Cooking Time: 20 minutes
Servings: 4
Ingredients:
- 1 whole river trout
- 1 teaspoon thyme
- ¼ diced yellow pepper
- ¼ diced green pepper
- 1 juiced lime
- ¼ diced red pepper
- 1 teaspoon oregano
- 1 teaspoon extra virgin olive oil
- 1 teaspoon black pepper

Directions:
1. Preheat the broiler/grill on high heat.
2. Lightly oil a baking tray.
3. Mix all the ingredients apart from the trout and lime.
4. Slice the trout lengthways (there should be an opening here from where it was gutted) and stuff the mixed ingredients inside.
5. Squeeze the lime juice over the fish and then place the lime wedges on the tray.
6. Place under the broiler on the baking tray and broil for 15-20

minutes or until fish is thoroughly cooked through and flakes easily.
7. Enjoy the dish as it is, or with a side helping of rice or salad.

Nutrition:
- Calories: 290
- Protein: 15 g
- Carbohydrates: 0 g
- Fat: 7 g
- Sodium (Na): 43 mg
- Potassium (K): 315 mg
- Phosphorus: 189 mg

150. Haddock & Buttered Leeks
Preparation Time: 5 minutes
Cooking Time: 15 minutes
Servings: 2
Ingredients:
- 1 tablespoon unsalted butter
- 1 sliced leek
- ¼ teaspoon black pepper
- 2 teaspoons chopped parsley
- 6 oz. haddock fillets
- ½ juiced lemon

Directions:
1. Preheat the oven to 375°F/Gas Mark 5.
2. Add the haddock fillets to baking or parchment paper and sprinkle with the black pepper.
3. Squeeze over the lemon juice and wrap into a parcel.
4. Bake the parcel on a baking tray for 10-15 minutes or until the fish is thoroughly cooked through.
5. Meanwhile, heat the butter over medium-low heat in a small pan.
6. Add the leeks and parsley and sauté for 5-7 minutes until soft.
7. Serve the haddock fillets on a bed of buttered leeks and enjoy!

Nutrition:
- Calories: 124 Protein: 15 g
- Carbohydrates: 0 g Fat: 7 g
- Sodium (Na): 161 mg
- Potassium (K): 251 mg
- Phosphorus: 220 mg

151. Thai Spiced Halibut
Preparation Time: 5 minutes
Cooking Time: 20 minutes
Servings: 2
Ingredients:
- 2 tablespoons coconut oil
- 1 cup white rice
- ¼ teaspoon black pepper
- ½ diced red chili
- 1 tablespoon fresh basil
- 2 pressed garlic cloves
- 4 oz. halibut fillet
- 1 halved lime
- 2 sliced green onions
- 1 lime leaf

Directions:
1. Preheat oven to 400°F/Gas Mark 5.
2. Add half of the ingredients into baking paper and fold into a parcel.
3. Repeat for your second parcel.
4. Add to the oven for 15-20 minutes or until fish is thoroughly cooked through.
5. Serve with cooked rice.

Nutrition:
- Calories: 311 Protein: 16 g
- Carbohydrates: 17 g Fat: 15 g
- Sodium (Na): 31 mg
- Potassium (K): 418 mg
- Phosphorus: 257 mg

152. Monk-Fish Curry

Preparation Time: 5 minutes
Cooking Time: 20 minutes
Servings: 2
Ingredients:
- 1 garlic clove
- 3 finely chopped green onions
- 1 teaspoon grated ginger
- 1 cup water.
- 2 teaspoons chopped fresh basil
- 1 cup cooked rice noodles
- 1 tablespoon coconut oil
- ½ sliced red chili
- 4 oz. Monkfish fillet
- ½ finely sliced stick lemongrass
- 2 tablespoons chopped shallots

Directions:
1. Slice the Monkfish into bite-size pieces.
2. Using a pestle and mortar or food processor, crush the basil, garlic, ginger, chili, and lemongrass to form a paste.
3. Heat the oil in a large wok or pan over medium-high heat and add the shallots.
4. Now add the water to the pan and bring to a boil.
5. Add the Monkfish, lower the heat, and cover to simmer for 10 minutes or until cooked through.
6. Enjoy with rice noodles and scatter with green onions to serve.

Nutrition:
- Calories: 249 Protein: 12 g
- Carbohydrates: 30 g
- Fat: 10 g
- Sodium (Na): 32 mg
- Potassium (K) 398 mg
- Phosphorus: 190 mg

153. Oregon Tuna Patties

Preparation Time: 10 minutes
Cooking Time: 15 minutes
Servings: 4
Ingredients:
- 1 (14.75-ounce) can tuna
- 2 tablespoons butter
- 1 medium onion, chopped
- 2/3 cup graham cracker crumbs
- 2 egg whites, beaten
- ¼ cup chopped fresh parsley
- 1 teaspoon dry mustard
- 3 tablespoons olive oil

Directions:
1. Drain the tuna, reserving 3/4 cup of the liquid. Flake the meat. Melt butter in a large skillet over medium-high heat. Add onion, and cook until tender.
2. In a medium bowl, combine the onions with the reserved tuna liquid, 1/3 of the graham cracker crumbs, egg whites, parsley, mustard, and tuna. Mix until well blended, then shape into six patties. Coat patties in remaining cracker crumbs.
3. Heat olive in a large skillet over medium heat. Cook patties until browned, then carefully turn and brown on the other side.

Nutrition:
- Calories: 204 Total Fat: 15.4 g
- Saturated Fat: 4.4 g
- Cholesterol: 74 mg
- Sodium: 111 mg
- Total Carbohydrates: 6.5 g
- Dietary Fiber: 0.9 g
- Total Sugar: 2 g Protein: 10.5 g
- Calcium: 21 mg Iron: 1 mg
- Potassium: 164 mg
- Phosphorus: 106 mg

154. Fish Chowder

Prep Time: 20 minutes
Cooking Time: 40 minutes
Servings: 4
Ingredients:
- 2 tablespoons butter
- 2 cups chopped onion
- 4 fresh mushrooms, sliced
- 1 stalk celery, chopped
- 4 cups chicken stock
- 2 pounds' cod, diced into ½ inch cubes
- ½ cup all-purpose flour
- 1/8 teaspoon Mrs. Dash salt-free seasoning, or to taste
- Ground black pepper to taste
- 2 (12 fluid ounce) cans soy milk

Directions:
1. In a large stockpot, melt 2 tablespoons butter over medium heat. Sauté onions, mushrooms, and celery in butter until tender.
2. Add chicken stock simmer for 10 minutes. Add cod, and simmer another 10 minutes.
3. Mix flour until smooth; stir into soup and simmer for 1 minute more. Season to taste with seasoning and pepper. Remove from heat, and stir in soy milk.

Nutrition:
- Calories: 171 Total Fat: 4.2 g
- Saturated Fat: 2.1 g
- Cholesterol: 32 mg
- Sodium: 810 mg
- Total Carbohydrates: 19.3 g
- Dietary Fiber: 2 g Total Sugar 3.9 g
- Protein: 14.1 g Calcium: 41 mg
- Iron: 2 mg Potassium: 204 mg
- Phosphorus: 106 mg

155. Broiled Sesame Cod

Preparation Time: 05 minutes
Cooking Time: 10 min
Servings: 4
Ingredients:
- ½ pounds' cod fillets
- 1 teaspoon butter, melted
- 1 teaspoon lemon juice
- 1 teaspoon dried basil
- 1 pinch ground black pepper
- 1 tablespoon sesame seeds

Directions:
1. Preheat the oven's broiler and set the oven rack about 6 inches from the heat source. Line a broiler pan with aluminum foil.
2. Place the cod fillets on the foil, and brush with butter. Season with lemon juice, basil, and black pepper; sprinkle with sesame seeds.
3. Broil the fish in the preheated broiler until the flesh turns opaque and white, and the fish flakes easily, about 10 minutes.

Nutrition:
- Calories: 67 Total Fat: 2.6 g
- Saturated Fat: 0.8 g
- Cholesterol: 30 mg
- Sodium 43 mg
- Total Carbohydrates: 0.6 g
- Dietary Fiber: 0.3 g
- Total Sugar 0 g
- Protein: 10.6 g
- Calcium 23 mg
- Iron 0 mg
- Potassium: 13 mg
- Phosphorus: 10 mg

156. Tuna Salad with Cranberries

Preparation Time: 10 minutes
Cooking Time: 0 minutes
Servings: 4
Ingredient:

- 2 (5 ounce) cans solid white tuna packed in water, drained
- 2 tablespoons mayonnaise
- 1/3 teaspoon dried dill weed
- 3 tablespoons dried cranberries

Directions:
1. Place the tuna in a bowl, and mash with a fork.
2. Mix in mayonnaise to evenly coat tuna. Mix in dill and cranberries.

Nutrition:
- Calories: 81
- Total Fat: 2.8 g
- Saturated Fat: 0.5 g
- Cholesterol: 15 mg
- Sodium: 74 mg
- Total Carbohydrates: 2.3 g
- Dietary Fiber: 0.2 g
- Total Sugar: 0.7 g
- Protein: 10.9 g
- Calcium: 8 mg
- Iron: 1 mg
- Potassium: 113 mg
- Phosphorus: 95 mg

157. Zucchini Cups with Dill Cream and Smoked Tuna

Preparation Time: 15 minutes
Cooking Time: 35 minutes
Servings: 4
Ingredients:

- 1 1/3 large Zucchini
- 4 ounces' cream cheese, softened
- 2 tablespoons chopped fresh dill
- 1 teaspoon lemon zest
- ½ teaspoon fresh lemon juice
- ¼ teaspoon ground black pepper
- 4 ounces smoked tuna, cut into 2-inch strips

Directions:
1. Trim ends from Zucchini and cut crosswise into 24 (3/4-inch-thick) rounds. Scoop a ½-inch-deep depression from one side of each round with a small melon-baller, forming little cups. Drain Zucchini, cup sides down, on paper towels for 15 minutes.
2. Beat cream cheese, chopped dill, lemon zest, lemon juice, and black pepper together in a bowl. Spoon ½ teaspoon cheese mixture into each Zucchini cup. Top each cup with 1 tuna strip.

Nutrition:
- Calories: 51
- Total Fat: 3.8 g
- Saturated Fat: 2.2 g
- Cholesterol: 13 mg
- Sodium: 219 mg
- Total Carbohydrates: 1.8 g
- Dietary Fiber: 0.3 g
- Total Sugar: 0.6 g
- Protein: 2.8 g
- Calcium: 24 mg
- Iron: 1 mg
- Potassium: 95 mg
- Phosphorus: 40 mg

158. Creamy Smoked Tuna Macaroni

Preparation Time: 15 minutes
Cooking Time: 25min
Servings: 4
Ingredients:

- 3 tablespoons olive oil
- ¼ onion, finely chopped
- 1 tablespoon all-purpose flour
- 1 teaspoon garlic powder
- 1 cup soy milk - ¼ cup cream cheese
- ½ cup frozen green peas, thawed and drained
- ¼ cup mushrooms
- 5 ounces smoked tuna, chopped
- ½ (16-ounce) package macaroni

Directions:

1. Bring a large pot of water to a boil. Add macaroni and cook for 8 to 10 minutes or until al dente; drain.
2. Heat oil in a large skillet over medium heat. Sauté onion in oil until tender.
3. Stir flour and garlic powder into the oil and onions. Gradually stir in milk. Heat to just below boiling point, and then gradually stir in cheese until the sauce is smooth. Stir in peas and mushrooms. Cook over low heat for 4 minutes.
4. Toss in smoked tuna, and cook for 2 more minutes. Serve over macaroni.

Nutrition:

- Calories: 147 Total Fat: 8.3 g
- Saturated Fat: 1.9 g
- Cholesterol: 14 mg Sodium: 979 mg
- Total Carbohydrates: 6.5 g
- Dietary Fiber: 0.8 g Total Sugar 1.9 g
- Protein: 11.4 g Calcium: 38 mg
- Iron: 1 mg Potassium: 160 mg
- Phosphorus: 100 mg

159. Asparagus and Smoked Tuna Salad

Preparation Time: 15 minutes
Cooking Time: 10 minutes
Servings: 4
Ingredients:

- ½ pound fresh asparagus, trimmed and cut into 1-inch pieces
- 1 heads lettuce, rinsed and torn
- ¼ cup frozen green peas, thawed
- 1/8 cup olive oil
- 1 tablespoon lemon juice
- ½ teaspoon Dijon mustard
- 1/8 teaspoon pepper
- 1/8 pound smoked tuna, cut into 1inch chunks

Directions:

1. Bring a pot of water to a boil. Place asparagus in the pot, and cook 5 minutes, just until tender. Drain, and set aside.
2. In a large bowl, toss together the asparagus, lettuce, peas, and tuna.
3. In a separate bowl, mix the olive oil, lemon juice, Dijon mustard, and pepper. Toss with the salad or serve on the side.

Nutrition:

- Calories: 87 Total Fat: 7 g
- Saturated Fat: 1.1 g
- Cholesterol: 3 mg
- Sodium: 298 mg
- Total Carbohydrates: 2.7 g
- Dietary Fiber: 1.1 g
- Total Sugar 1 g Protein: 3.8 g
- Calcium: 16 mg Iron: 1 mg
- Potassium: 134 mg
- Phosphorus: 104 mg

160. Spicy Tuna Salad Sandwiches
Preparation Time: 15 minutes
Cooking Time: 0 minutes
Servings: 2
Ingredients:
- 1 (8 ounces) can tuna, undrained
- ¼ cucumber, chopped
- 2 tablespoons light mayonnaise
- 1 tablespoon vinegar
- 1 teaspoon red chili paste
- 4 slices white bread, toasted

Directions:
1. Put tuna into a bowl and use a fork to flake and mix with the can's liquid. Mix cucumber with the tuna.
2. Stir mayonnaise, vinegar, chili paste, and bowl; add hot sauce and adjust to taste. Pour mayonnaise mixture over the salmon mixture and stir to coat. Spoon onto toasted bread to make sandwiches.

Nutrition:
- Calories: 189
- Total Fat: 7.6 g
- Saturated Fat: 1.1 g
- Cholesterol: 28 mg
- Sodium: 326 mg
- Total Carbohydrates: 15.6 g
- Dietary Fiber: 2.1 g
- Total Sugar 3.4 g
- Protein: 15.1 g
- Calcium: 60 mg
- Iron: 1 mg
- Potassium: 119 mg
- Phosphorus: 109 mg

161. Spanish Tuna
Preparation Time: 20 minutes
Cooking Time: 15 minutes
Servings: 4
Ingredients:
- 1 tablespoon olive oil
- ¼ cup finely chopped onion
- 2 tablespoons chopped fresh garlic
- ¼ cup basil chopped
- 1 dash black pepper
- 1 dash cayenne pepper
- 1 dash paprika
- 6 (4-ounce) fillets tuna fillets

Directions:
1. Heat olive oil in a large skillet over medium heat.
2. Cook and stir onions and garlic until onions are slightly tender; careful not to burn the garlic.
3. Season with black pepper, cayenne pepper, basil, and paprika.
4. Cook fillets in sauce over medium heat for 5 to 8 minutes, or until easily flaked with a fork. Serve immediately.

Nutrition:
- Calories: 130
- Total Fat: 4.6 g
- Saturated Fat: 0.5 g
- Cholesterol: 55 mg
- Sodium: 71 mg
- Total Carbohydrates: 2.2 g
- Dietary Fiber: 0.3 g
- Total Sugar 0.4 g
- Protein: 20.4 g
- Calcium: 10 mg
- Iron: 0 mg
- Potassium: 31 mg
- Phosphorus: 46 mg

162. Fish with Vegetables

Preparation Time: 30 minutes
Cooking Time: 60 minutes
Servings: 4
Ingredients:
- 1 egg white, beaten
- ¼ cup all-purpose flour
- Black pepper to taste
- 1-pound firm salmon fillets, cut into 1 ½-inch pieces
- ½ cup olive oil, divided
- 1 onion, cut in half and thinly sliced
- 1 carrot, peeled and coarsely grated
- ½ large turnips, peeled and coarsely grated
- ½ leek coarsely grated
- 1 cup water

Directions:
1. Place egg white and flour in 2 shallow bowls. Season egg white with pepper. Dip fish pieces first in the beaten egg, then dredge in the flour.
2. Heat ¼ cup olive oil in a deep skillet over medium heat until hot. Add fish in batches and fry on both sides until golden, 5 to 8 minutes per batch. Remove fish from skillet and set aside.
3. Heat remaining ¼ cup oil in a separate skillet and cook onions until soft and translucent, about 5 minutes. Add carrots, turnips, and leek; mix well. Add water and season with pepper. Cover and simmer on low heat until vegetables are soft, about 30 minutes. Check and add more water if the mixture becomes too dry.
4. Layer vegetables and fried fish in a 10-inch round serving dish, starting and ending with vegetables.

Nutrition:
- Calories: 358
- Total Fat: 30.1 g
- Saturated Fat: 6 g
- Cholesterol: 57 mg
- Sodium: 45 mg
- Total Carbohydrates: 14.7 g
- Dietary Fiber: 2.2 g
- Total Sugar 3.3 g
- Protein: 8.2 g
- Calcium: 38 mg
- Iron: 1 mg
- Potassium: 281 mg
- Phosphorus: 161 mg

163. Creamy Crab over Salmon

Preparation Time: 10 minutes
Cooking Time: 15 minutes
Servings: 4
Ingredients:
- ¼ cup olive oil, divided
- 2 (4 ounce) fillets salmon
- 1 teaspoon dried oregano
- 1 pinch ground white pepper
- 1 3/4 cups soy milk
- 4 ounces' fresh crabmeat
- 1 teaspoon lemon juice

Directions:
1. Heat a small amount of olive oil in a non-stick skillet over medium heat. Season salmon with oregano and white pepper; cook in skillet until the flesh flakes easily with a fork, 7 to 10 minutes per side.
2. While fish cooks, whisk the remaining olive oil and the soy milk together in a saucepan over medium-low heat; cook, stirring regularly, until it thickens, 3 to 5 minutes. Remove the saucepan from heat and stir crab meat into the sauce.

3. Transfer cooked cod to plates and spoon sauce over the fish.

Nutrition:
- Calories: 258 Total Fat: 16.5 g
- Saturated Fat: 2.5 g
- Cholesterol: 40 mg
- Sodium: 395 mg
- Total Carbohydrates: 11.4 g
- Dietary Fiber: 1 g Total Sugar 6.1 g
- Protein: 17.3 g Calcium: 37 mg
- Iron: 1 mg Potassium: 160 mg
- Potassium: 120 mg

164. Fish Tacos

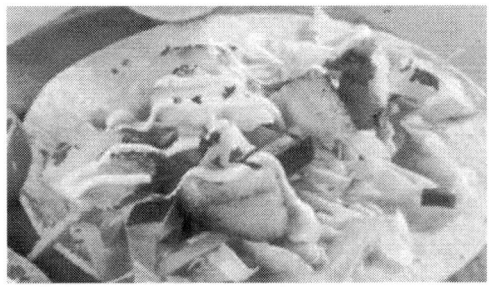

Preparation Time: 10 minutes
Cooking Time: 35 minutes
Servings: 6
Ingredients:
- 1½ cup of cabbage
- ½ cup of red onion
- ½ bunch of cilantro
- 1 garlic clove
- 2 limes
- 1 pound of cod fillets
- ½ teaspoon of ground cumin
- ½ teaspoon of chili powder
- ¼ teaspoon of black pepper
- 1 tablespoon of olive oil
- ½ cup of mayonnaise
- ¼ cup of sour cream
- 2 tablespoons of milk
- 12 (6-inch) corn tortillas

Directions:
1. Shred the cabbage, chop the onion and cilantro, and mince the garlic. Set aside
2. Use a dish to place in the fish fillets, then squeeze half a lime juice over the fish. Sprinkle the fish fillets with the minced garlic, cumin, black pepper, chili powder, and olive oil. Turn the fish filets to coat with the marinade, then refrigerate for about 15 to 30 minutes
3. Prepare salsa Blanca by mixing the mayonnaise, milk, sour cream, and the other half of the lime juice. Stir to combine, then place in the refrigerator to chill
4. Broil in oven, and cover the broiler pan with aluminum foil. Broil the coated fish fillets for about 10 minutes or until the flesh becomes opaque and white and flakes easily. Remove from the oven, slightly cool, and then flake the fish into bigger pieces
5. Heat the corn tortillas in a pan, one at a time until it becomes soft and warm, then wrap in a dish towel to keep them warm
6. To assemble the tacos, place a piece of the fish on the tortilla, topping with the salsa blanca, cabbage, cilantro, red onion, and the lime wedges.

Serve with hot sauce if you desire

Nutrition:
- Calories 363 Protein 18g
- Carbohydrates 30g Fat 19g
- Cholesterol 40mg
- Sodium 194mg
- Potassium 507mg
- Phosphorus 327mg Fiber 4.3g

165. Jambalaya

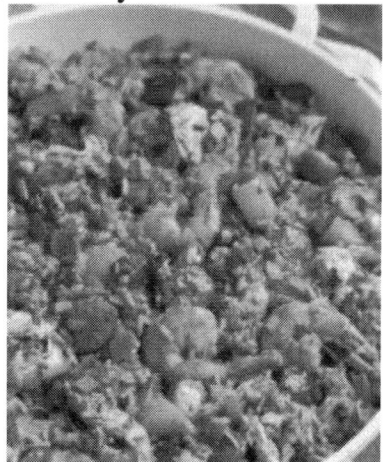

Preparation Time: 10 minutes
Cooking Time: 1 hour and 15 minutes
Servings: 12
Ingredients:

- 2 cups of onion
- 1 cup of bell pepper
- 2 garlic cloves
- 2 cups of uncooked converted brown rice
- ½ teaspoon of black pepper
- 8 ounces of canned low-sodium tomato sauce
- 2 cups of low-sodium beef broth
- 2 pounds of raw shrimp
- ½ cup of unsalted margarine

Directions:

1. Preheat oven to 350° F
2. Chop the onion, bell pepper, garlic, then peel the shrimp
3. Combine and mix all the ingredients in a large bowl except the margarine
4. Pour into a 9 x 13-inch baking dish and evenly spread out
5. Slice the margarine, placing over the top of the ingredients
6. Cover with foil or lid, and bake for about 1 hour 15 minutes

Serve hot.
Nutrition:

- Calories 294
- Protein 20g
- Carbohydrates 31g
- Fat 10g
- Cholesterol 137mg
- Sodium 186mg
- Potassium 300mg
- Phosphorus 197mg
- Fiber 0.8g

166. Asparagus Shrimp Linguini

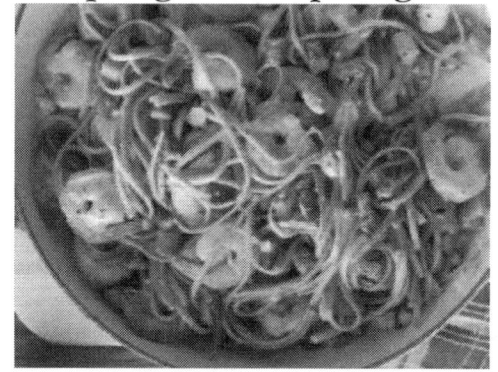

Preparation Time: 10 minutes
Cooking Time: 35 minutes
Servings: 1 ½ cup
Ingredients:

- 8 ounces of uncooked linguini
- 1 tablespoon of olive oil
- 1 ¾ cups of asparagus
- ½ cup of unsalted butter
- 2 garlic cloves
- 3 ounces of cream cheese
- 2 tablespoons of fresh parsley
- ¾ teaspoon of dried basil
- ⅔ cup of dry white wine
- ½ pound of peeled and cooked shrimp

Directions:
1. Preheat oven to 350° F
2. Cook the linguini in boiling water until it becomes tender, then drain
3. Place the asparagus on a baking sheet, then spread two tablespoons of oil over the asparagus. Bake for about 7 to 8 minutes or until it is tender
4. Remove baked asparagus from the oven and place it on a plate. Cut the asparagus into pieces of medium-sized once cooled
5. Mince the garlic and chop the parsley
6. Melt ½ cup of butter in a large skillet with the minced garlic
7. Stir in the cream cheese, mixing as it melts
8. Stir in the parsley and basil, then simmer for about 5 minutes. Mix either in boiling water or dry white wine, stirring until the sauce becomes smooth
9. Add the cooked shrimp and asparagus, then stir and heat until it is evenly warm

Toss the cooked pasta with the sauce and serve

Nutrition:
- Calories 544
- Protein 21g
- Carbohydrates 43g
- Fat 32g
- Cholesterol 188mg
- Sodium 170mg
- Potassium 402mg
- Phosphorus 225mg
- Fiber 2.4g

167. Tuna Noodle Casserole

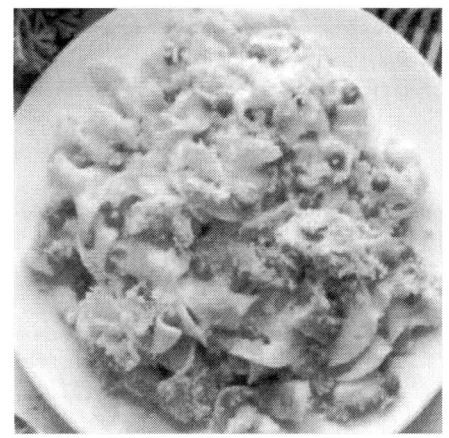

Preparation Time: 10 minutes
Cooking Time: 35 minutes
Servings: 2

Ingredients:
- 2 ounces of wide uncooked egg noodles
- 5 ounces of canned tuna in water
- ½ cup of sour cream
- ¼ cup of cottage cheese
- ½ cup of fresh sliced mushrooms
- ½ cup of frozen green peas
- 1 tablespoon of unsalted butter
- ¼ cup of unseasoned bread crumbs

Directions:
1. Preheat oven to 350° F
2. Boil egg noodles based on the package instructions and drain. Also, drain and flake the tuna
3. Combine and mix the sour cream, cottage cheese, mushrooms, tuna, and peas in a medium bowl
4. Stir the drained noodle into the tuna mixture, and place in a small casserole dish that has been sprayed with a non-stick cooking spray
5. Melt butter, stir into the bread crumbs, then sprinkle over the mixture of noodles in step 4

6. Bake for about 20 to 25 minutes or until the bread crumbs start to brown

Divide into two and serve

Nutrition:
- Calories 415
- Protein 22g
- Carbohydrates 39g
- Fat 19g
- Cholesterol 88mg
- Sodium 266mg
- Potassium 400mg
- Phosphorus 306mg
- Fiber 3.2g

168. Oven-Fried Southern Style Catfish

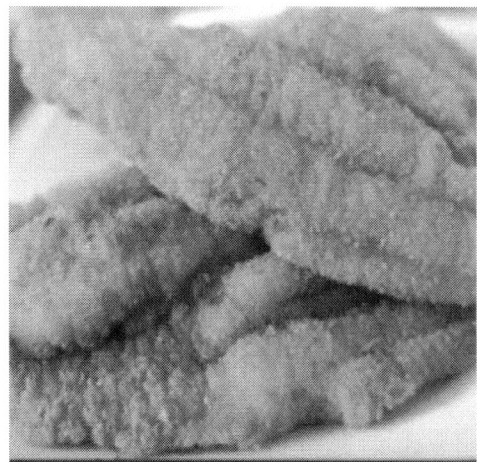

Preparation Time: 10 minutes
Cooking Time: 35 minutes
Servings: 4
Ingredients:
- 1 egg white
- ½ cup of all-purpose flour
- ¼ cup of cornmeal
- ¼ cup of panko bread crumbs
- 1 teaspoon of salt-free Cajun seasoning
- 1 pound of catfish fillets

Directions:
1. Heat oven to 450° F
2. Use cooking spray to spray a non-stick baking sheet
3. Using a bowl, beat the egg white until very soft peaks are formed. Don't over-beat
4. Use a sheet of wax paper and place the flour over it
5. Using a different sheet of wax paper to combine and mix the cornmeal, panko and the Cajun seasoning
6. Cut the catfish fillet into four pieces, then dip the fish in the flour, shaking off the excess
7. Dip coated fish in the egg white, rolling into the cornmeal mixture
8. Place the fish on the baking pan. Repeat with the remaining fish fillets
9. Use cooking spray to spray over the fish fillets. Bake for about 10 to 12 minutes or until the sides of the fillets become browned and crisp

Nutrition:
- Calories 250
- Protein 22g
- Carbohydrates 19g
- Fat 10g
- Cholesterol 53mg
- Sodium 124mg
- Potassium 401mg
- Phosphorus 262mg
- Fiber 1.2g

169. Cilantro-Lime Cod

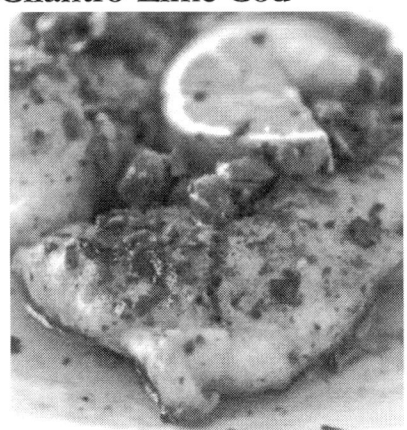

Preparation Time: 10 minutes
Cooking Time: 35 minutes
Servings: 4
Ingredients:
- ½ cup of mayonnaise
- ½ cup of fresh chopped cilantro
- 2 tablespoon of lime juice
- 1 pound of cod fillets

Directions:
1. Combine and mix the mayonnaise, cilantro, and lime juice in a medium bowl, remove ¼ cup to another bowl and put aside. To be served as fish sauce
2. Spread the remaining mayonnaise mixture over the cod fillets
3. Use cooking spray to spray a large skillet, then heat over medium-high heat
4. Place in the cod fillets, and cook for about 8 minutes or until the fish becomes firm and moist, turning just once

Serve with the ¼ cilantro-lime sauce

Nutrition:
- Calories 292
- Protein 20g
- Carbohydrates 1g
- Fat 23g
- Cholesterol 57mg
- Sodium 228mg
- Potassium 237mg
- Phosphorus 128mg
- Calcium 14mg

170. Shrimp Quesadilla

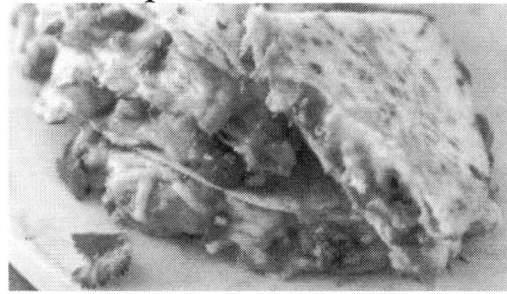

Preparation Time: 15 minutes
Cooking Time: 10 minutes
Servings: 2
Ingredients:
- 5 ounces of raw shrimp
- 2 tablespoons of cilantro
- 1 tablespoon of lemon juice
- ¼ teaspoon of ground cumin
- ⅛ teaspoon of cayenne pepper
- 2 flour burrito-sized tortillas
- 2 tablespoons of sour cream
- 4 teaspoons of salsa
- 2 tablespoons of shredded jalapeno cheddar cheese

Directions:
1. Peel the shrimp, rinse, and then cut into pieces of bite-size. Dice the cilantro
2. Use a zip-lock bag to combine and mix the cilantro, lemon juice, cumin, and cayenne pepper to make the marinade. Add the pieces of shrimp and put aside to marinate for about 5 minutes

3. Heat a skillet over medium heat and add the shrimp with the marinade. Stir-fry for about 1 to 2 minutes or until the shrimp is orange in color. Remove the skillet from heat and spoon out the shrimp, leaving marinade
4. Add the sour cream to the skillet with the leftover marinade. Stir to mix
5. Use a large skillet or microwave to heat the tortillas, then spread two teaspoons of salsa over each tortilla. Top with ½ of the shrimp mixture, sprinkling with one tablespoon of cheddar cheese
6. Spoon out one tablespoon of the sour cream mixture from step 4 on top of the shrimp, fold the tortilla into half, turning over in skillet to heat, then remove from the pan. Repeat the same process with the second tortilla and with the remaining shrimp, cheese and marinade

Cut each of the tortillas into four pieces, and serve

Nutrition:
- Calories 318
- Protein 20g
- Carbohydrates 26g
- Fat 15g
- Cholesterol 118mg
- Sodium 398mg
- Potassium 276mg
- Phosphorus 243mg
- Fiber 1.2g

CHAPTER 6:

Meat

171. Pork Souvlaki
Preparation Time: 20 minutes
Cooking Time: 12 minutes
Servings: 8
Ingredients:
- 3 tablespoons olive oil
- 2 tablespoons lemon juice
- 1 teaspoon minced garlic
- 1 tablespoon chopped fresh oregano
- ¼ teaspoon ground black pepper
- 1 pound pork leg, cut into 2-inch cubes

Directions:
1. In a bowl, stir together the lemon juice, olive oil, garlic, oregano, and pepper.
2. Add the pork cubes and toss to coat.
3. Place the bowl in the refrigerator, covered, for 2 hours to marinate.
4. Thread the pork chunks onto 8 wooden skewers that have been soaked in water.
5. Preheat the barbecue to medium-high heat.
6. Grill the pork skewers for about 12 minutes, turning once, until just cooked through but still juicy.

Nutrition:
- Calories: 95 Fat: 4 g
- Carb: 0 g Phosphorus: 125 mg
- Potassium: 230 mg
- Sodium: 29 mg
- Protein: 13 g

172. Open-Faced Beef Stir-Up
Preparation Time: 10 minutes
Cooking Time: 10 minutes
Servings: 6
Ingredients:
- ½ pound 95% lean ground beef
- ½ cup chopped sweet onion
- ½ cup shredded cabbage
- ¼ cup herb pesto
- 6 hamburger buns, bottom halves only

Directions:
1. Sauté the beef and onion for 6 minutes or until the beef is cooked.
2. Add the cabbage and sauté for 3 minutes more.
3. Stir in pesto and heat for 1 minute.
4. Divide the beef mixture into 6 portions and serve each on the bottom half of a hamburger bun, open-face.

Nutrition:
- Calories: 120 Fat: 3 g
- Phosphorus: 106 mg
- Potassium: 198 mg
- Sodium: 134 mg
- Protein: 11 g

173. Grilled Steak with Cucumber Salsa

Preparation Time: 20 minutes
Cooking Time: 15 minutes
Servings: 4
Ingredients:
For the salsa:

- ¼ cup boiled and diced red bell pepper
- 1 cup chopped English cucumber
- 1 scallion both green and white parts, chopped
- 2 tablespoons chopped fresh cilantro
- Juice of 1 lime

For the steak:

- Olive oil
- Beef tenderloin steaks 4(3-ounce), room temperature
- Freshly ground black pepper

Directions:

1. In a bowl, to make the salsa combine the lime juice, cilantro, scallion, bell pepper, and cucumber. Set aside.
2. To make the steak: Preheat a barbecue to medium heat.
3. Rub the steaks all over with oil and season with pepper.
4. Grill the steaks for about 5 minutes per side for medium-rare, or until the desired state.
5. Serve the steaks topped with salsa.

Nutrition:

- Calories: 130 Fat: 6 g
- Carb: 1 g Phosphorus: 186 mg
- Potassium: 272 mg
- Sodium: 39 mg
- Protein: 19 g

174. Beef Brisket

Preparation Time: 10 minutes
Cooking Time: 3 ½ hours
Servings: 6
Ingredients:

- 12 ounces trimmed chuck roast
- 2 cloves garlic
- 1 tablespoon thyme
- tablespoon rosemary
- 1 tablespoon mustard
- ¼ cup extra virgin olive oil
- 1 teaspoon black pepper
- 1 onion, diced
- 1 cup carrots, peeled and sliced
- 2 cups low salt stock

Directions:

1. Preheat the oven to 300F.
2. Soak vegetables in warm water.
3. Make a paste by mixing the thyme, mustard, rosemary, and garlic. Then mix in the oil and pepper.
4. Add the beef to the dish.
5. Pour the mixture over the beef into a dish.
6. Place the vegetables onto the bottom of the baking dish around the beef.
7. Cover and roast for 3 hours or until tender.
8. Uncover the dish and continue to cook for 30 minutes in the oven.
9. Serve.

Nutrition:

- Calories: 303 Fat: 25 g
- Carb: 7 g
- Phosphorus: 376 mg
- Potassium: 246 mg
- Sodium: 44 mg
- Protein: 18 g

175. Lamb Shoulder with Zucchini and Eggplant

Preparation Time: 10 minutes
Cooking Time: 4 to 5 hours
Servings: 2
Ingredients:
- 6 ounces lean lamb shoulder
- 2 zucchinis, cubed
- 1 eggplant, cubed
- 1 teaspoon black pepper
- 2 tablespoons extra virgin olive oil
- 1 tablespoon basil
- 1 tablespoon oregano
- 2 cloves garlic, chopped

Directions:
1. Preheat the oven to its highest setting.
2. Soak the vegetables in warm water.
3. Trim any fat from the lamb shoulder.
4. Rub the lamb with 1 tablespoon olive oil, pepper, and herbs.
5. Line a baking tray with the rest of the olive oil, garlic, zucchini, and eggplant.
6. Add the lamb shoulder and cover with foil.
7. Turn the oven down to 325F and add the dish into the oven.
8. Cook for 4 to 5 hours, remove and rest.
9. Slice the lamb and then serve with the vegetables.

Nutrition:
- Calories: 478 Fat: 31 g
- Carb: 13 g
- Phosphorus: 197 mg
- Potassium: 414 mg
- Sodium: 84 mg
- Protein: 33 g

176. Beef Chili

Preparation Time: 10 minutes
Cooking Time: 30 minutes
Servings: 2
Ingredients:
- 1 onion, diced
- 1 red bell pepper, diced
- 2 cloves garlic, minced
- 6 ounces lean ground beef
- 1 teaspoon chili powder
- 1 teaspoon oregano
- 2 tablespoons extra virgin olive oil
- 1 cup water - 1 cup rice
- 1 tablespoon fresh cilantro, to serve

Directions:
1. Soak vegetables in warm water.
2. Bring a pan of water to a boil and add rice for 20 minutes.
3. Meanwhile, add the oil to a pan and heat on medium-high heat.
4. Add the pepper, onions, and garlic and sauté for 5 minutes until soft.
5. Remove and set aside.
6. Add the beef to the pan and stir until browned.
7. Add the vegetables back into the pan and stir.
8. Now add the chili powder and herbs and water, cover, and turn the heat down a little to simmer for 15 minutes.
9. Meanwhile, drain the rice and add the lid, and steam while the chili is cooking. Serve hot with the fresh cilantro sprinkled over the top.

Nutrition:
- Calories: 459 Fat: 22 g
- Carb: 36 g Phosphorus: 332 mg
- Potassium: 360 mg Protein: 22 g

177. Skirt Steak Glazed with Bourbon

Preparation Time: 30 minutes
Cooking Time: 50 minutes (1 hour additional)
Servings: 8

Ingredients:

- Bourbon glaze
- ¼ cup shallots (diced)
- 3 tablespoons unsalted butter (chilled)
- 1 cup Bourbon
- ¼ cup dark brown sugar
- 2 tablespoons Dijon mustard
- 1 tablespoon black pepper
- Skirt steak
- 2 tablespoons grapeseed oil
- ½ teaspoon dried oregano
- ½ teaspoon smoked paprika
- 1 teaspoon black pepper
- 1 tablespoon red wine vinegar
- 2 pounds skirt steak

Directions:

1. Start by preparing the bourbon glaze. For this, you will need to take a small saucepan and place it over a medium-high flame.
2. Add in 1 tablespoon of butter and toss in the shallots. Stir-fry until they turn brown.
3. Reduce the heat to the minimum and remove the saucepan from the stove. Pour in the bourbon and stir thoroughly. Return the saucepan to the stove.
4. Let this cook on a low flame for about 15 minutes. Make sure the glaze reduces to one-third.
5. Stir in the dark sugar, black pepper, and Dijon mustard. Keep stirring until the glaze becomes bubbly.
6. Turn off the flame and add in about 2 tablespoons of cold butter. Keep stirring to incorporate with the sauce.
7. Now prepare the skirt steak. To do this, take a gallon-sized zip-lock bag and add in the grapeseed oil, dried oregano, smoked paprika, black pepper, and red wine vinegar. Mix well.
8. Now add in the steaks and shake well. Allow the steaks to sit in the marinade for about 45 minutes.
9. Remove the steaks from the zip-lock bag. Set aside.
10. Heat the grill and place the steaks on it. Cook for about 20 minutes.
11. Once done, remove the steak and place it on a baking tray. Let it rest for about 10 minutes before serving.
12. Slice the steaks and drizzle the glaze on top. Place the tray in the broiler for 5 minutes. Serve hot!

Nutrition:

- Protein: 24 g
- Carbohydrates: 8 g
- Fat: 22 g
- Cholesterol: 93 mg
- Sodium: 152 mg
- Potassium: 283 mg
- Phosphorus: 171 mg
- Calcium: 22 mg
- Fiber: 0.5 g

178. Beef Pot Roast

Preparation Time: 20 minutes
Cooking Time: 1 hour
Servings: 3
Ingredients:
- Round bone roast
- 2 - 4 pounds' chuck roast

Directions:
1. Trim off excess fat.
2. Place a tablespoon of oil in a large skillet and heat to medium.
3. Roll pot roast in flour and brown on all sides in a hot skillet.
4. After the meat gets a brown color, reduce heat to low.
5. Season with pepper and herbs and add ½ cup of water.
6. Cook slowly for 1½ hours or until it looks ready.

Nutrition:
- Calories: 157
- Protein: 24 g
- Fat: 13 g
- Carbs: 0 g
- Phosphorus: 204 mg
- Sodium (Na): 50 mg

179. Grilled Lamb Chops

Preparation Time: 10 minutes
Cooking Time: 6 minutes
Servings: 1
Ingredients:
- 1 tablespoon fresh ginger, grated
- 4 garlic cloves, chopped roughly
- 1 teaspoon ground cumin
- ½ teaspoon red chili powder
- Salt and freshly ground black pepper, to taste
- 1 tablespoon essential olive oil
- 1 tablespoon fresh lemon juice
- 8 lamb chops, trimmed

Directions:
1. In a bowl, mix all ingredients except chops.
2. With a hand blender, blend till a smooth mixture is formed.
3. Add chops and coat generously with mixture.
4. Refrigerate to marinate overnight.
5. Preheat the barbecue grill till hot. Grease the grill grate.
6. Grill the chops for approximately 3 minutes per side.
7. Serve when done.

Nutrition:
- Calories: 227
- Fat: 12 g
- Phosphorus: 36 mg
- Potassium: 194 mg
- Sodium: 31 mg
- Carbohydrates: 1 g
- Fiber: 0 g
- Protein: 30 g.

180. Lamb & Pineapple Kebabs

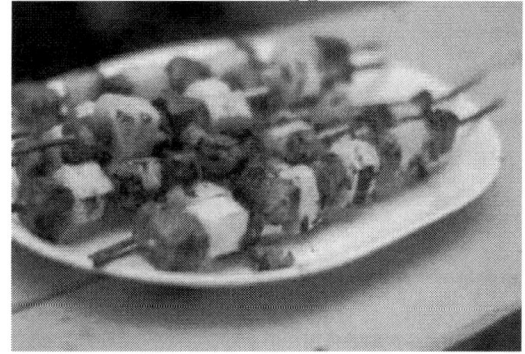

Preparation Time: 15 minutes
Cooking Time: 10 minutes
Servings: 1
Ingredients:
- 1 large pineapple, cubed into 1½-inch size, divided

- 1 (½-inch) piece fresh ginger, chopped
- 2 garlic cloves, chopped
- Salt, to taste
- 16-24-ounce lamb shoulder steak, trimmed and cubed into 1½-inch size
- Fresh mint leaves coming from a bunch
- Ground cinnamon, to taste

Directions:
1. Add about one half of pineapple, ginger, garlic, and salt and pulse till smooth in a blender.
2. Transfer the mixture into a large bowl.
3. Add chops and coat generously with the mixture.
4. Refrigerate to marinate for about 1-2 hours.
5. Preheat the grill to medium heat. Grease the grill grate.
6. Thread lam, remaining pineapple and mint leaves onto pre-soaked wooden skewers.
7. Grill the kebabs for approximately 10 minutes, turning occasionally.
8. Serve when done.

Nutrition:
- Calories: 482
- Fat: 16 g
- Phosphorus: 36 mg
- Potassium: 194 mg
- Sodium: 31 mg
- Carbohydrates: 22 g
- Fiber: 5 g Protein: 377 g.

181. Baked Meatballs & Scallions

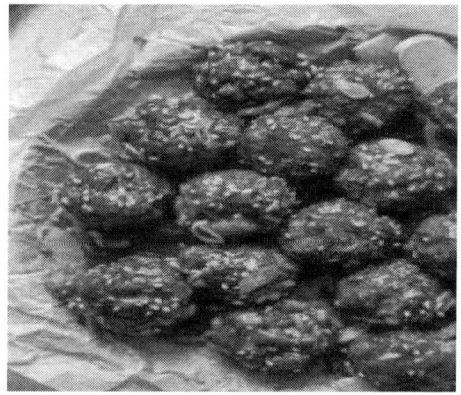

Preparation Time: 20 minutes
Cooking Time: 35 minutes
Servings: 1
Ingredients:
For Meatballs:

- 1 lemongrass stalk, outer skin peeled and chopped
- 1 (1½-inch) piece fresh ginger, sliced
- 3 garlic cloves, chopped
- 1 cup fresh cilantro leaves, chopped roughly
- ½ cup fresh basil leaves, chopped roughly
- 2 tablespoons plus 1 teaspoon fish sauce
- 2 tablespoons water
- 2 tablespoons fresh lime juice
- ½ pound lean ground pork
- 1-pound lean ground lamb
- 1 carrot, peeled and grated
- 1 organic egg, beaten

For Scallions:
- 16 stalks scallions, trimmed
- 2 tablespoons coconut oil, melted
- Salt, to taste
- ½ cup water

Directions:
1. Preheat the oven to 3750 F. Grease a baking dish.
2. In a blender, add lemongrass, ginger, garlic, fresh herbs, fish sauce, water, and lime juice and pulse till chopped finely.
3. Transfer the mixture to a bowl with the remaining ingredients and mix well.
4. Make about 1-inch balls from the mixture.
5. Arrange the balls into the prepared baking dish in a single layer.
6. In another rimmed baking dish, arrange scallion stalks in a single layer.
7. Drizzle with coconut oil and sprinkle with salt.
8. Pour water into the baking dish, then, with foil paper, cover it tightly.
9. Bake the scallion for around a half-hour.
10. Bake the meatballs for approximately 30-35 minutes.
11. Serve the meatballs and scallion when done.

Nutrition:
- Calories: 432
- Fat: 13 g
- Phosphorus: 45 mg
- Potassium: 78 mg
- Sodium: 34 mg
- Carbohydrates: 25 g
- Fiber: 8 g
- Protein: 40 g.

182. Pork with Bell Pepper

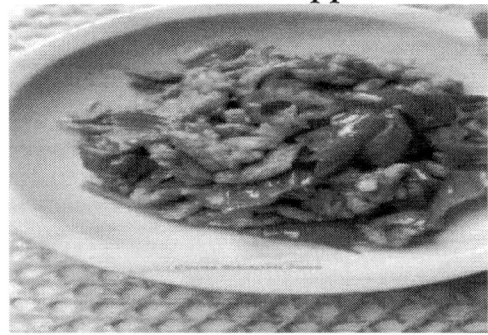

Preparation Time: 15 minutes
Cooking Time: 13 minutes
Servings: 1
Ingredients:
- 1 tablespoon fresh ginger, chopped finely
- 4 garlic cloves, chopped finely
- 1 cup fresh cilantro, chopped and divided
- ¼ cup plus 1 tablespoon olive oil, divided
- 1-pound tender pork, trimmed, sliced thinly
- 2 onions, sliced thinly
- 1 green bell pepper, seeded and sliced thinly
- 1 tablespoon fresh lime juice

Directions:
1. In a substantial bowl, mix ginger, garlic, ½ cup of cilantro, and ¼ cup of oil.
2. Add pork and coat with mixture generously.
3. Refrigerate to marinate for a couple of hours.
4. Heat a big skillet on medium-high heat.
5. Add pork mixture and stir fry for approximately 4-5 minutes.
6. Transfer the pork right into a bowl.

7. In the same skillet, heat the remaining oil on medium heat.
8. Add onion and sauté for approximately 3 minutes.
9. Stir in bell pepper and stir fry for about 3 minutes.
10. Stir in pork, lime juice, and remaining cilantro and cook for about 2 minutes.
11. Serve hot.

Nutrition:
- Calories: 429
- Fat: 19 g
- Phosphorus: 36 mg
- Potassium: 57 mg
- Sodium: 31 mg
- Carbohydrates: 26 g
- Fiber: 9 g
- Protein: 35 g.

183. Pork with Pineapple

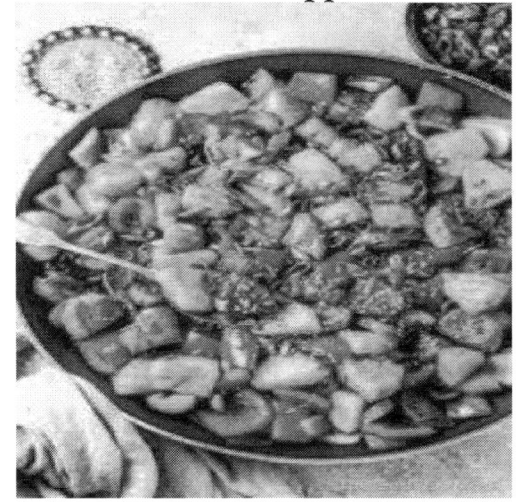

Preparation Time: 15 minutes
Cooking Time: 14 minutes
Servings: 1
Ingredients:
- 2 tablespoons coconut oil
- 1½ pound pork tenderloin, trimmed and cut into bite-sized pieces
- 1 onion, chopped
- 2 minced garlic cloves
- 1 (1-inch) piece fresh ginger, minced
- 20-ounce pineapple, cut into chunks
- 1 large red bell pepper, seeded and chopped
- ¼ cup fresh pineapple juice
- ¼ cup coconut aminos
- Salt and freshly ground black pepper, to taste

Directions:
1. In a substantial skillet, melt coconut oil on high heat.
2. Add pork and stir fry for approximately 4-5 minutes.
3. Transfer the pork into a bowl.
4. In the same skillet, heat the remaining oil on medium heat.
5. Add onion, garlic, and ginger and sauté for around 2 minutes.
6. Stir in pineapple and bell pepper and stir fry for around 3 minutes.
7. Stir in pork, pineapple juice, and coconut aminos and cook for around 3-4 minutes.
8. Serve hot.

Nutrition:
- Calories: 431
- Fat: 10 g
- Phosphorus: 36 mg
- Potassium: 64 mg
- Sodium: 30 mg
- Carbohydrates: 22 g
- Fiber: 8 g
- Protein: 33 g.

184. Pork Chili

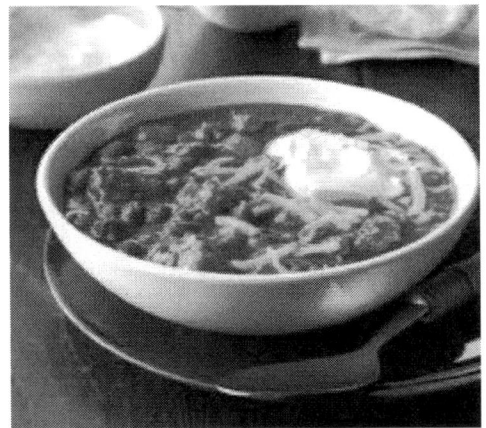

Preparation Time: 15 minutes
Cooking Time: 1 hour
Servings: 1
Ingredients:

- 2 tablespoons extra-virgin organic olive oil
- 2-pound ground pork
- 1 medium red bell pepper, seeded and chopped
- 1 medium onion, chopped
- 5 garlic cloves, chopped finely
- 1 (2-inch) part of hot pepper, minced
- 1 tablespoon ground cumin
- 1 teaspoon ground turmeric
- 3 tablespoon chili powder
- ½ teaspoon chipotle chili powder
- Salt and freshly ground black pepper, to taste
- 1 cup chicken broth
- 2 medium Bok choy heads, sliced

Directions:

1. In a sizable pan, heat oil on medium heat.
2. Add pork and stir fry for about 5 minutes.
3. Add bell pepper, onion, garlic, hot pepper, and spices and stir fry for approximately 5 minutes.
4. Add broth and convey with a boil.
5. Stir in Bok choy and cook, covered for approximately twenty minutes.
6. Uncover and cook for approximately 20 minutes to half an hour.

Nutrition:

- Calories: 402
- Fat: 9 g
- Phosphorus: 20 mg
- Potassium: 156 mg
- Sodium: 34 mg
- Carbohydrates: 18 g
- Fiber: 6 g
- Protein: 32 g.

185. Ground Pork with Water Chestnuts

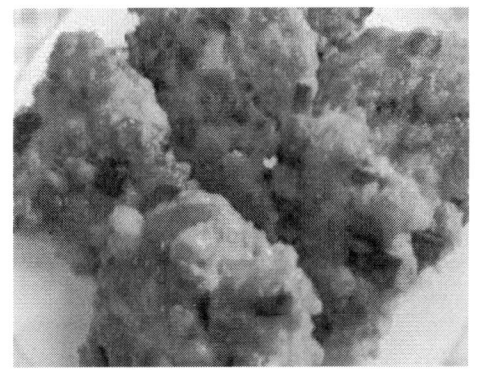

Preparation Time: 15 minutes
Cooking Time: 12 minutes
Servings: 1
Ingredients:

- 1 tablespoon plus 1 teaspoon coconut oil
- 1 tablespoon fresh ginger, minced
- 1 bunch scallion (white and green parts separated), chopped
- 1-pound lean ground pork
- Salt, to taste
- 1 tablespoon 5-spice powder

- 1 (18-ounce) can water chestnuts, drained and chopped
- 1 tablespoon organic honey
- 2 tablespoons fresh lime juice

Directions:
1. In a big heavy-bottomed skillet, heat oil on high heat.
2. Add ginger and scallion whites and sauté for approximately ½-1½ minutes.
3. Add pork and cook for approximately 4-5 minutes.
4. Drain the extra fat from the skillet.
5. Add salt and 5-spice powder and cook for approximately 2-3 minutes.
6. Add scallion greens and remaining ingredients and cook, stirring continuously for about 1-2 minutes.

Nutrition:
- Calories: 520
- Fat: 30 g
- Phosphorus: 20 mg
- Potassium: 120 mg
- Sodium: 9 mg
- Carbohydrates: 37 g
- Fiber: 4 g
- Protein: 25 g.

186. Hearty Meatloaf

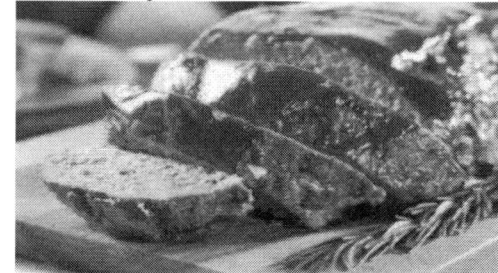

Preparation Time: 10 minutes
Cooking Time: 45-50 minutes
Servings: 1
Ingredients:
- 1 large egg
- 2 tablespoons chopped fresh basil
- 1 teaspoon chopped fresh thyme
- 1 teaspoon chopped fresh parsley
- ¼ teaspoon black pepper (ground)
- 1 pound 95% lean ground beef
- ½ cup breadcrumbs
- ½ cup chopped sweet onion
- 1 teaspoon white vinegar
- ¼ teaspoon garlic powder
- 1 tablespoon brown sugar

Directions:
1. Preheat an oven to 350°F. Grease a loaf pan (9X5-inch) with some cooking spray.
2. In a mixing bowl, add beef, breadcrumbs, onion, egg, basil, thyme, parsley, and black pepper. Combine to mix.
3. Add the mixture to the pan.
4. Take another mixing bowl; add brown sugar, vinegar, and garlic powder. Combine to mix well.
5. Add brown sugar mixture over the meat mixture.
6. Bake for about 50 minutes until golden brown.
7. Serve warm.

Nutrition:
- Calories: 118
- Fat: 3 g
- Phosphorus: 127 mg
- Potassium: 203 mg
- Sodium: 106 mg
- Carbohydrates: 8 g
- Protein: 12 g.

187. Chicken with Mushrooms

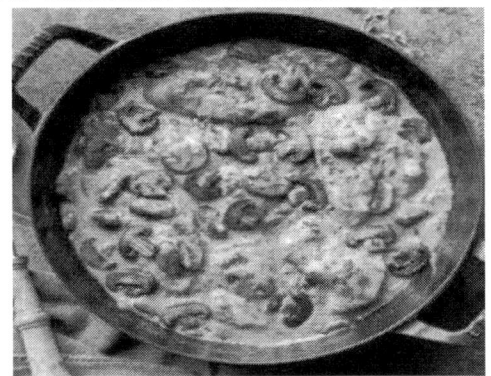

Preparation Time: 15 minutes
Cooking Time: 45 minutes
Servings: 2
Ingredients:

- 2 tablespoons light sour cream
- ¼ cup all-purpose flour
- 1 cup no salt added chicken broth
- 1 tablespoon Dijon mustard
- ¼ teaspoon dried thyme
- 4 chicken breasts
- 1½ cups mushrooms, quartered
- 1 tablespoon non-hydrogenated margarine
- Fresh ground pepper and chopped fresh parsley, to taste
- 3 chopped green onions

Directions:

1. Mix 2 tablespoon of chicken broth, mustard, sour cream, and 2 teaspoon flour. Set aside.
2. Sprinkle chicken with pepper and thyme. Dredge in flour.
3. Melt margarine on medium-low heat in a large non-stick pan. Cook chicken for 15-20 minutes per side. Remove from heat and keep warm.
4. Add mushrooms to another pan. Increase the heat and boil for 3 minutes.
5. Add sour cream mixture and green onions and cook until thickened.
6. Pour over chicken. Garnish with parsley and pepper.

Nutrients:

- Protein: 25.4 g
- Phosphorus: 29 mg
- Potassium: 142 mg
- Sodium: 17 mg
- Carbohydrates: 5 g
- Fat: 4 g
- Calories: 161.

CHAPTER 7:

Poultry

188. Roasted Citrus Chicken
Preparation Time: 20 minutes
Cooking Time: 60 minutes
Servings: 8
Ingredients:
- 1 tablespoon olive oil
- 2 cloves garlic, minced
- 1 teaspoon Italian seasoning
- ½ teaspoon black pepper
- 8 chicken thighs
- 2 cups chicken broth, reduced-sodium
- 3 tablespoons lemon juice
- ½ large chicken breast for 1 chicken thigh

Directions:
1. Warm oil in a huge skillet.
2. Include garlic and seasonings.
3. Include chicken bosoms and dark-colored all sides.
4. Spot chicken in the moderate cooker and include the chicken soup.
5. Cook on LOW heat for 6 to 8 hours
6. Include lemon juice toward the part of the bargain time.

Nutrition:
- Calories: 265
- Fat: 19 g
- Protein: 21 g
- Carbs: 1 g

189. Chicken with Asian Vegetables
Preparation Time: 10 minutes
Cooking Time: 20 minutes
Servings: 8
Ingredients:
- 2 - tablespoons canola oil
- 6 - boneless chicken breasts
- 1 - cup low-sodium chicken broth
- 3 - tablespoons reduced-sodium soy sauce
- ¼ - teaspoon crushed red pepper flakes
- 1 - garlic clove, crushed
- 1 - can (8ounces) water chestnuts, sliced and rinsed (optional)
- ½ - cup sliced green onions
- 1 - cup chopped red or green bell pepper
- 1 - cup chopped celery
- ¼ - cup cornstarch
- ⅓ - cup water
- 3 - cups cooked white rice
- ½ - large chicken breast for 1 chicken thigh

Directions:
1. Warm oil in a skillet and dark-colored chicken on all sides.
2. Add chicken to the slow cooker with the remainder of the fixings aside from cornstarch and water.
3. Spread and cook on LOW for 6 to 8 hours.

4. Following 6-8 hours, independently blend cornstarch and cold water until smooth. Gradually include into the moderate cooker.
5. At that point, turn on high for about 15 minutes until thickened. Don't close the top on the moderate cooker to enable steam to leave.
6. Serve Asian blend over rice.

Nutrition:
- Calories: 415
- Fat: 20 g
- Protein: 20 g
- Carbs: 36 g

190. Chicken Adobo

Preparation Time: 10 minutes
Cooking Time: 1 hour and 40 minutes
Servings: 6
Ingredients:
- 4 medium yellow onions, halved and thinly sliced
- 4 medium garlic cloves, smashed and peeled
- 1 (5-inch) piece fresh ginger, cut into 1-inch pieces
- 1 bay leaf
- 3 pounds bone-in chicken thighs
- 3 tablespoons reduced-sodium soy sauce
- ¼ cup rice vinegar (not seasoned)
- 1 tablespoon granulated sugar
- ½ teaspoon freshly ground black pepper

Directions:
1. Spot the onions, garlic, ginger, and narrows leaf in an even layer in the slight cooker.
2. Take out and do away with the pores and skin from the chicken.
3. Organize the hen in an even layer over the onion mixture.
4. Whisk the soy sauce, vinegar, sugar, and pepper collectively in a medium bowl and pour it over the fowl.
5. Spread and prepare dinner on LOW for 8 hours
6. Evacuate and take away the ginger portions and inlet leaf.
7. Present with steamed rice.

Nutrition:
- Calories: 318
- Fat: 9 g
- Protein: 14 g
- Carbs: 44 g

191. Chicken and Veggie Soup

Preparation Time: 15 minutes
Cooking Time: 25 minutes
Servings: 8
Ingredients:
- 4 - cups cooked and chopped chicken
- 7 - cups reduced-sodium chicken broth
- 1 - pound frozen white corn
- 1 - medium onion diced
- 4 - cloves garlic minced
- 2 - carrots peeled and diced
- 2 - celery stalks chopped
- 2 - teaspoons oregano
- 2 - teaspoon curry powder
- ½ - teaspoon black pepper

Directions:
1. Include all fixings into the moderate cooker.
2. Cook on LOW for 8 hours

3. Serve over cooked white rice.

Nutrition:
- Calories: 220
- Fat: 7 g
- Protein: 24 g
- Carbs: 19 g

192. Turkey Sausages

Preparation Time: 10 Minutes
Cooking Time: 10 minutes
Servings: 2
Ingredients:
- ¼ teaspoon salt
- 1/8 teaspoon garlic powder
- 1/8 teaspoon onion powder
- 1 teaspoon fennel seed
- 1 pound 7% fat ground turkey

Directions:
1. Press the fennel seed and put together turkey with fennel seed, garlic and onion powder, and salt in a small cup.
2. Cover the bowl and refrigerate overnight.
3. Prepare the turkey with seasoning into different portions with a circle form and press them into patties ready to be cooked.
4. Cook at medium heat until browned.
5. Cook it for 1 to 2 minutes per side and serve them hot. Enjoy!

Nutrition:
- Calories: 55
- Protein: 7 g
- Sodium: 70 mg
- Potassium: 105 mg
- Phosphorus: 75 mg

193. Smoky Turkey Chili

Preparation Time: 5 minutes
Cooking Time: 45 minutes
Servings: 8
Ingredients:
- 12-ounce lean ground turkey
- ½ red onion, chopped
- 2 cloves garlic, crushed and chopped
- ½ teaspoon of smoked paprika
- ½ teaspoon of chili powder
- ½ teaspoon of dried thyme
- ¼ cup reduced-sodium beef stock
- ½ cup of water
- 3 wheat tortillas

Directions:
1. Brown the ground beef in a dry skillet over medium-high heat.
2. Add in the red onion and garlic.
3. Sauté the onion until it goes clear.
4. Transfer the contents of the skillet to the slow cooker.
5. Add the remaining ingredients and simmer on low for 30–45 minutes.
6. Slice tortillas and gently toast under the broiler until slightly crispy.
7. Serve on top of the turkey chili.

Nutrition:
Per serving:
- Calories: 93.5
- Protein: 8 g
- Carbohydrates: 3 g
- Fat: 5.5 g
- Cholesterol: 30.5 mg
- Sodium: 84.5 mg
- Potassium: 142.5 mg
- Phosphorus: 92.5 mg
- Calcium: 29 mg Fiber: 0.5 g

194. Rosemary Chicken

Preparation Time: 10 Minutes
Cooking Time: 10 minutes
Servings: 2
Ingredients:
- 2 zucchinis
- 1 carrot
- 1 teaspoon dried rosemary
- 4 chicken breasts
- ½ bell pepper
- ½ red onion
- 8 garlic cloves
- Olive oil
- ¼ tablespoon ground pepper

Directions:
1. Prepare the oven and preheat it at 375 °F (or 200°C).
2. Slice both zucchini and carrots and add bell pepper, onion, garlic, and put everything adding oil in a 13" x 9" pan.
3. Spread the pepper over everything and roast for about 10 minutes.
4. Meanwhile, lift the chicken skin and spread black pepper and rosemary on the flesh.
5. Remove the vegetable pan from the oven and add the chicken, returning it to the oven for about 30 more minutes. Serve and enjoy!

Nutrition:
- Calories: 215
- Protein: 28 g
- Sodium: 105 mg
- Potassium: 580 mg
- Phosphorus: 250 mg

195. Herbs and Lemony Roasted Chicken

Preparation Time: 15 minutes
Cooking Time: 1 ½ hours
Servings: 8
Ingredients:
- ½ teaspoon ground black pepper
- ½ teaspoon mustard powder
- ½ teaspoon salt
- 1 3-lb whole chicken
- 1 teaspoon garlic powder
- 2 lemons
- 2 tablespoons. olive oil
- 2 teaspoons. Italian seasoning

Directions:
1. In a small bowl, mix well black pepper, garlic powder, mustard powder, and salt.
2. Rinse chicken well and slice off giblets.
3. In a greased 9 x 13 baking dish, place chicken and add 1 ½ teaspoon of seasoning made earlier inside the chicken and rub the remaining seasoning around the chicken.
4. In a small bowl, mix olive oil and juice from 2 lemons. Drizzle over chicken.
5. Bake chicken in a preheated 350oF oven until juices run clear, around 1 ½ hours. Every once in a while, baste the chicken with its juices.

Nutrition:
- Calories per serving: 190
- Carbs: 2 g Protein: 35 g
- Fats: 9 g
- Phosphorus: 341 mg
- Potassium: 439 mg
- Sodium: 328 mg

196. Ground Chicken & Peas Curry

Preparation Time: 15 minutes
Cooking Time: 6-10 minutes
Servings: 3-4
Ingredients:
For Marinade:

- 3 tablespoons essential olive oil
- 2 bay leaves
- 2 onions, grinded to some paste
- ½ tablespoon garlic paste
- ½ tablespoon ginger paste
- 1 tablespoon ground cumin
- 1 tablespoon ground coriander
- 1 teaspoon ground turmeric
- 1 teaspoon red chili powder
- Salt, to taste
- 1-pound lean ground chicken
- 2 cups frozen peas
- 1½ cups water
- 1-2 teaspoons garam masala powder

Directions:
1. In a deep skillet, heat oil on medium heat.
2. Add bay leaves and sauté for approximately half a minute.
3. Add onion paste and sauté for approximately 3-4 minutes.
4. Add garlic and ginger paste and sauté for around 1-1½ minutes.
5. Add spices and cook, occasionally stirring for about 3-4 minutes.
6. Stir in chicken and cook for about 4-5 minutes.
7. Stir in peas and water and bring to a boil on high heat.
8. Reduce the heat to low and simmer approximately 5-8 minutes or till the desired doneness.
9. Stir in garam masala and remove from heat.
10. Serve hot.

Nutrition:
- Calories: 450
- Fat: 10 g
- Carbohydrates: 19 g
- Fiber: 6 g
- Protein: 38 g

197. Chicken Meatballs Curry

Preparation Time: 20 minutes
Cooking Time: 25 minutes
Servings: 3-4
Ingredients:
For Meatballs:

- 1-pound lean ground chicken
- 1 tablespoon onion paste
- 1 teaspoon fresh ginger paste
- 1 teaspoon garlic paste
- 1 green chili, chopped finely
- 1 tablespoon fresh cilantro leaves, chopped
- 1 teaspoon ground coriander
- ½ teaspoon cumin seeds
- ½ teaspoon red chili powder
- ½ teaspoon ground turmeric
- Salt, to taste

For Curry:

- 3 tablespoons extra-virgin olive oil
- ½ teaspoon cumin seeds
- 1 (1-inch) cinnamon stick
- 3 whole cloves
- 3 whole green cardamoms
- 1 whole black cardamom
- 2 onions, chopped
- 1 teaspoon fresh ginger, minced
- 1 teaspoon garlic, minced

- 2 teaspoons ground coriander
- 1 teaspoon garam masala powder
- ½ teaspoon ground nutmeg
- ½ teaspoon red chili powder
- ½ teaspoon ground turmeric
- Salt, to taste
- 1 cup water
- Chopped fresh cilantro, for garnishing

Directions:
1. For meatballs in a substantial bowl, add all ingredients and mix till well combined.
2. Make small equal-sized meatballs from the mixture.
3. In a big deep skillet, heat oil on medium heat.
4. Add meatballs and fry approximately 3-5 minutes or till browned from all sides.
5. Transfer the meatballs to a bowl.
6. In the same skillet, add cumin seeds, cinnamon stick, cloves, green cardamom, and black cardamom and sauté for approximately 1 minute.
7. Add onions and sauté for around 4-5 minutes.
8. Add ginger and garlic paste and sauté for approximately 1 minute.
9. Add tomato and spices and cook, crushing with the back of a spoon for approximately 2-3 minutes.
10. Add water and meatballs and provide to a boil.
11. Reduce heat to low.
12. Simmer for approximately 10 minutes.
13. Serve hot with all the garnishing of cilantro.

Nutrition:
- Calories: 421
- Fat: 8 g
- Carbohydrates: 18 g
- Fiber: 5 g
- Protein: 34 g

CHAPTER 8:

Soup

198. Chicken and Corn Soup
Preparation Time: 30 minutes
Cooking Time: 3 hours
Servings: 12
Ingredients:
- 4lb roasting chicken
- 3 cup medium-size flat noodles, uncooked
- 2 cans unsalted corn, drained
- 1 tbsp. dried parsley
- ¼ tsp. black pepper
- 14 cup water

Directions:
1. Cook the chicken in a large pot with 8 cups of water.
2. Reserve the broth and after cooling the chicken, chop meat into small pieces.
3. Cook noodles according to package instructions, drain and set aside.
4. Place 6 cups of water, 6 cups of broth, cooked chicken, cooked noodles, corn, parsley, and pepper into a large stockpot.
5. Bring to a boil, simmer, and serve.

Nutrition:
- Calories: 222
- Total Carbs: 17 g
- Net Carbs: 15 g
- Protein: 25 g
- Potassium: 303 mg
- Phosphorous: 212 mg

199. Pumpkin Bacon Soup
Preparation Time: 10 minutes
Cooking Time: 15 minutes
Servings: 2
Ingredients:
- 2 teaspoons ground ginger
- 1 teaspoon cinnamon
- 1 cup applesauce
- 3 ½ cups low sodium chicken broth
- 1 onion, chopped
- 1 slice of bacon
- 1 29-ounce can pumpkin
- Pepper, to taste
- ½ cup light sour cream

Directions:
1. Take a medium-large cooking pot; add bacon and cook on both sides over medium heat until crispy for 4-5 minutes.
2. Remove bacon fat.
3. Add ginger, applesauce, chicken broth, pumpkin, and black pepper to taste. Stir mixture.
4. Over low heat, simmer the mixture for about 10 minutes. Season to taste.
5. Take off heat and mix in the cream.

6. Serve warm.

Nutrition:
- Calories: 256
- Fat: 9 g
- Phosphorus: 192 mg
- Potassium: 746 mg
- Sodium: 148 mg
- Carbohydrates: 33 g
- Protein: 8 g

200. Classic Chicken Soup
Preparation Time: 10 minutes
Cooking Time: 35 minutes
Servings: 2
Ingredients:
- 2 teaspoons minced garlic
- 2 celery stalks, chopped
- 1 tablespoon unsalted butter
- ½ sweet onion, diced
- 1 carrot, diced
- 4 cups of water
- 1 teaspoon chopped fresh thyme
- 2 cups chopped cooked chicken breast
- 1 cup chicken stock
- Black pepper (ground), to taste
- 2 tablespoons chopped fresh parsley

Directions:
1. Take a medium-large cooking pot, heat oil over medium heat.
2. Add onion and stir-cook until become translucent and softened.
3. Add garlic and stir-cook until you become fragrant.
4. Add celery, carrot, chicken, chicken stock, and water.
5. Boil the mixture.
6. Over low heat, simmer the mixture for about 25-30 minutes until veggies are tender.
7. Mix in thyme and cook for 2 minutes. Season to taste with black pepper.
8. Serve warm with parsley on top.

Nutrition:
- Calories: 135
- Fat: 6 g
- Phosphorus: 122 mg
- Potassium: 208 mg
- Sodium: 74 mg
- Carbohydrates: 3 g
- Protein: 15 g

201. Beef Okra Soup
Preparation Time: 10 minutes
Cooking Time: 45 minutes
Servings: 5
Ingredients:
- ½ cup okra
- ½ teaspoon basil
- ½ cup carrots, diced
- 3 ½ cups water
- 1-pound beef stew meat
- 1 cup raw sliced onions
- ½ cup green peas
- 1 teaspoon black pepper
- ½ teaspoon thyme
- ½ cup corn kernels

Directions:
1. Take a medium-large cooking pot, heat oil over medium heat.
2. Add water, beef stew meat, black pepper, onions, basil, thyme, and stir-cook for 40-45 minutes until meat is tender.
3. Add all veggies. Over low heat, simmer the mixture for about 20-

25 minutes. Add more water if needed.
4. Serve soup warm.

Nutrition:
- Calories: 187
- Fat: 12 g
- Phosphorus: 119 mg
- Potassium: 288 mg
- Sodium: 59 mg
- Carbohydrates: 7 g
- Protein: 11 g

202. Chicken Pasta Soup
Preparation Time: 10 minutes
Cooking Time: 20 minutes
Servings: 6
Ingredients:
- 2 tablespoons orzo (tiny pasta)
- 1 tablespoon dry white wine
- 1 14-ounce low sodium chicken broth
- ½ teaspoon Italian seasoning
- 1 large shallot, chopped
- 1 small zucchini, diced
- 8 ounces chicken tenders
- 1 tablespoon extra-virgin olive oil

Directions:
1. Take a medium saucepan or skillet, add oil. Heat over medium heat.
2. Add chicken and stir-cook for 3 minutes until evenly brown. Set aside.
3. In the pan, add zucchini, Italian seasoning, and shallot. Stir-cook until veggies are softened.
4. Add wine, broth, and orzo.
5. Boil the mixture.

6. Over low heat, cover, and simmer the mixture for about 3 minutes.

Nutrition:
- Calories: 103
- Fat: 3 g
- Phosphorus: 125 mg
- Potassium: 264 mg
- Sodium: 84 mg
- Carbohydrates: 6 g
- Protein: 12 g

203. Cream of Watercress Soup
Preparation Time: 15 minutes
Cooking Time: 1 hour 15 minutes
Servings: 4
Ingredients:
- 6 garlic cloves
- ½ teaspoon olive oil
- 1 teaspoon unsalted butter
- ½ sweet onion, chopped
- 4 cups chopped watercress
- ¼ cup chopped fresh parsley
- 3 cups water
- ¼ cup heavy cream
- 1 tablespoon freshly squeezed lemon juice
- Freshly ground black pepper

Directions:
1. Preheat the oven to 400°F. Set your garlic on a sheet of foil. Drizzle with olive oil and fold the foil into a little packet. Place the packet on a pie plate and roast the garlic for about 20 minutes or very soft.
2. Switch off the oven and set your garlic to cool. Add your butter to melt in a saucepan on medium heat. Sauté the onion for about 4

minutes or until soft. Add the watercress and parsley; sauté 5 minutes. Stir in the water and roasted garlic pulp. Allow boiling, then switch the heat to low.

3. Simmer the soup for about 20 minutes or until the vegetables are soft. Cool the soup for about 5 minutes, then purée in batches in a food processor (or use a large bowl and a handheld immersion blender), along with the heavy cream.
4. Transfer the soup to the pot, and set over low heat until warmed through. Add the lemon juice and season with pepper.

Nutrition:
- Calories: 97
- Fat: 8 g
- Carbs: 5 g
- Phosphorus: 46 mg
- Potassium: 198 mg
- Sodium: 23 mg
- Protein: 2 g

204. Curried Cauliflower Soup
Preparation Time: 20 minutes
Cooking Time: 30 minutes
Servings: 6
Ingredients:
- 1 teaspoon unsalted butter
- 1 small sweet onion, chopped
- 2 teaspoons minced garlic
- 1 small head cauliflower, cut into small florets
- 3 cups water, or more to cover the cauliflower
- 2 teaspoons curry powder
- ½ cup light sour cream
- 3 tablespoons chopped fresh cilantro

Directions:
1. In a large saucepan, heat the butter over medium-high heat and sauté the onion and garlic for about 3 minutes or until softened. Add the cauliflower, water, and curry powder.
2. Bring the soup to a boil, then reduce the heat to low and simmer for about 20 minutes or until the cauliflower is tender. Pour the soup into a food processor and purée until it is smooth and creamy (or use a large bowl and a handheld immersion blender).
3. Transfer the soup back into a saucepan and stir in the sour cream and cilantro. Heat the soup on medium-low for about 5 minutes or until warmed through.

Nutrition:
- Calories: 33 Fat: 2 g
- Carbs: 4 g
- Phosphorus: 30 mg
- Potassium: 167 mg
- Sodium: 22 mg
- Protein: 1 g

205. Asparagus Lemon Soup
Preparation Time: 10 minutes
Cooking Time: 25 minutes
Servings: 4 servings
Ingredients:
- 1-pound asparagus
- 2 tablespoons extra-virgin olive oil

- ½ sweet onion, chopped
- 4 cups low-sodium chicken stock
- ½ cup Homemade Rice Milk or unsweetened store-bought rice milk
- Freshly ground black pepper
- Juice of 1 lemon

Directions:
1. Cut the asparagus tips from the spears and set aside. In a small stockpot over medium heat, heat the olive oil. Add the onion and cook, stirring frequently for 3 to 5 minutes, until it softens. Add the stock and asparagus stalks, and bring to a boil.
2. Reduce the heat and simmer until the asparagus is tender, about 15 minutes. Transfer to a blender or food processor, and carefully purée until smooth. Return to the pot, add the asparagus tips, and simmer until tender, about 5 minutes. Add the rice milk, pepper, and lemon juice, and stir until heated through. Serve.

Nutrition:
- Calories: 145
- Fat: 9 g
- Carbs: 13 g
- Protein: 8 g
- Phosphorus: 143 mg
- Potassium: 497 mg
- Sodium: 92 mg

CHAPTER 9:

Salad

206. Hawaiian Chicken Salad
Preparation Time: 5 minutes
Cooking Time: 30 minutes
Ingredients:
- 1 ½ cups of chicken breast, cooked, chopped
- 1 cup pineapple chunks
- 1 ¼ cups lettuce iceberg, shredded
- ½ cup celery, diced
- ½ cup mayonnaise
- 1/8 tsp (dash) Tabasco sauce
- 2 lemon juice
- ¼ tsp black pepper

Directions:
1. Combine the cooked chicken, pineapple, lettuce, and celery in a medium bowl. Just set aside.
2. In a small bowl, make the dressing. Mix the mayonnaise, Tabasco sauce, pepper, and lemon juice.
3. Use the chicken mixture to add the dressing and stir until well mixed.

Nutrition:
- Power: 310 g Protein: 16.8 g
- Carbohydrates: 9.6 g
- Fibbers: 1.1 g Fat: 23.1 g
- Sodium: 200 mg
- Potassium: 260 mg
- Phosphorus: 134 mg

207. Grated Carrot Salad with Lemon-Dijon Vinaigrette
Preparation Time: 15 minutes
Cooking Time: 10 minutes
Servings: 8
Ingredients:
- 9 small carrots (14 cm), peeled
- 2 tbsp. ½ teaspoon Dijon mustard - 1 C. lemon juice
- 2 tbsp. extra virgin olive oil
- 1-2 tsp. honey (to taste)
- ¼ tsp. salt
- ¼ tsp. freshly ground pepper (to taste) - 2 tbsp. chopped parsley
- 1 green onion, thinly sliced

Directions:
1. Grate the carrots in a food processor.
2. In a salad bowl, mix Dijon mustard, lemon juice, honey, olive oil, salt, and pepper. Add the carrots, fresh parsley, and green onions. Stir to coat well. Cover and refrigerate until ready to be served.

Nutrition: Energy: 61 g Proteins: 1 g
- Carbohydrates: 7 g Fibbers: 1 g
- Total Fat: 4 g Sodium: 88 mg
- Phosphorus: 22 mg
- Potassium: 197 mg

208. Tuna Macaroni Salad
Preparation Time: 5 minutes
Cooking Time: 25 minutes
Servings: 10
Ingredients:
- 1 ½ cups Uncooked Macaroni
- 1 170 g Can of tuna in water
- ¼ cup Mayonnaise
- 2 medium celery stalks, diced
- 1 Tbsp. Lemon Pepper Seasoning

Directions:
1. Cook the pasta and let it cool in the refrigerator.
2. Drain the tuna in a colander and rinse it with cold water.
3. Add the tuna and celery once the macaroni has cooled.
4. Stir in mayonnaise and sprinkle with lemon seasoning. Mix well. Serve cold.

Nutrition:
- Power: 136 g
- Protein: 8.0 g
- Carbohydrates: 18 g
- Fibbers: 0.8 g
- Fat: 3.6 g
- Sodium: 75 mg
- Potassium: 124 mg
- Phosphorus: 90 mg

209. Couscous Salad
Preparation Time: 5 minutes
Cooking Time: 5 minutes
Servings: 5
Ingredients:
- 3 cups of water
- ½ tsp. cinnamon tea
- ½ tsp. cumin tea
- 1 tsp. honey soup
- 2 tbsp. lemon juice
- 3 cups quick-cooking couscous
- 2 tbsp. tea of olive oil
- 1 green onion,
- Finely chopped 1 small carrot, finely diced
- ½ red pepper,
- Finely diced fresh coriander

Directions:
1. Stir in the water with the cinnamon, cumin, honey, and lemon juice and bring to a boil. Put the couscous in it, cover it, and remove it from the heat. To swell the couscous, stir with a fork. Add the vegetables, fresh herbs, and olive oil. It is possible to serve the salad warm or cold.

Nutrition:
- Energy: 190 g
- Protein: 6 g
- Carbohydrates: 38 g
- Fibbers: 2 g
- Total Fat: 1 g
- Sodium: 4 mg
- Phosphorus: 82 mg
- Potassium: 116 mg

210. Fruity Zucchini Salad
Preparation Time: 5 minutes
Cooking Time: 5 minutes
Servings: 4
Ingredients:
- 400 g zucchini
- 1 small onion
- 4 tbsp. olive oil
- 100 g pineapple preserve, drained
- Salt, paprika
- Thyme

Directions:
1. Dice the onions and sauté in the oil until translucent.
2. Cut the zucchini into slices and add. Season with salt, paprika, and thyme.
3. Let cool and mix with the cut pineapple.

Nutrition:
- Energy: 150
- Protein: 2 g
- Fat: 10 g
- Carbohydrates: 10 g
- Dietary Fibbers: 2 g
- Potassium: 220 mg
- Calcium: 38 mg
- Phosphate: 24 mg

211. Cucumber Salad, Pulled Through Slowly

Preparation Time: 5 minutes
Cooking Time: 5 minutes
Servings: 4
Ingredients:
- 1 cucumber
- 1 tbsp. salt
- 100 ml of water
- 100 ml white wine vinegar
- 2 tbsp. cane sugar
- 5 peppercorns, crushed
- ½ teaspoon cinnamon
- ½ teaspoon of allspice
- 1 teaspoon chili powder
- 1 teaspoon ginger powder

Directions:
1. Wash the cucumber and cut it into thin slices, put them in a bowl, sprinkle with salt and stir, shake well so that the salt gets everywhere. Then let it steep for half an hour.
2. Meanwhile, in a saucepan, mix water, vinegar, sugar, pepper, cinnamon, allspice, chili, ginger, and bring to the boil once, then let cool again with the lid closed.
3. Rinse the lettuce slices and pour off the water. If necessary, dry in a towel. Add the pot's dressing to the salad slices and let everything sit in the fridge for a day.

Nutrition:
- Energy: 49
- Protein: 1 g
- Carbohydrates: 5 g
- Potassium: 234 mg
- Sodium: 500 mg
- Calcium: 34 mg
- Phosphate: 21 mg

212. Tortellini Salad

Preparation Time: 5 minutes
Cooking Time: 10 minutes
Servings: 4
Ingredients:
- 200 g tortellini with meat filling
- 100 g red peppers
- 1 tomato
- 1 clove of garlic
- Salt pepper
- Fresh basil, some leaves
- 3 tbsp. rapeseed oil
- 1 tbsp. white wine vinegar

Directions:
1. Cook the tortellini in salted water according to the instructions on the packet and drain.
2. Finely dice the pepper and garlic and sweat in the rapeseed oil. Add the vinegar and spices and pour over the tortellini. Cut the

tomato into small pieces and mix in. mix with the fresh basil and season to taste.

Nutrition:
- Energy: 161 Protein: 4 g
- Fat: 9 g
- Carbohydrates: 18 g
- Dietary Fibbers: 3 g
- Potassium: 173 mg
- Phosphate: 80 mg

213. Farmer's Salad
Preparation Time: 5 minutes
Cooking Time: 5 minutes
Servings: 2
Ingredients:
- 60 g mixed leaf salads
- 100 g red pepper, diced
- 200 g green beans
- 60 g feta cheese
- 1 tbsp. wine vinegar
- 1 tbsp. diced onions
- Salt, pepper, sugar
- 2 tbsp. olive oil

Directions:
1. Mix vinegar with onions, oil, and spices and mix with the salad.
2. Cut the sheep's cheese into cubes and serve with the salad. It goes well with baguette or flatbread with herb butter.

Nutrition:
- Energy: 187 Protein: 8 g
- Fat: 16 g
- Carbohydrates: 4 g
- Dietary Fibbers: 5 g
- Potassium: 396 mg
- Calcium: 188 mg
- Phosphate: 170 mg

214. Chicken and Asparagus Salad with Watercress
Preparation Time: 5 minutes
Cooking Time: 40 minutes
Servings: 4
Ingredients:
- 100 g spring onions (0.5 bunch)
- 100 g green asparagus
- 600 g chicken breast fillet (4 chicken breast fillets)
- Salt
- Pepper
- 1 small lime
- 1 clove of garlic
- 6 tbsp. honey
- 1 tbsp. grainy mustard
- 5 tbsp. olive oil
- 100 g watercress

Directions:
1. The spring onions are cleaned and washed and then cut into thin rings.
2. The woody ends of the asparagus are cut off. Wash and pat the asparagus to dry. Halve the sticks and, with a peeler, cut the halves lengthwise into thin slices.
3. Wash the fillets of chicken, pat them dry with kitchen paper, and cut them into strips. With salt and pepper, season.
4. Trim the lime in half for the dressing and squeeze out the juice. Peel the garlic and dice it. Mix the mustard, 3 tablespoons of lime juice, and 3 tablespoons of oil with the honey. With salt and pepper, season.
5. In a large non-stick pan, heat the remaining oil and stir-fry the

meat over high heat for about 5 minutes.
6. In a bowl, add the chicken, spring onions, and asparagus. Mix in the dressing and allow the salad too steep for 10 minutes or so.
7. Meanwhile, wash the cress and shake it dry. Pluck the leaves, chop coarsely as desired, and spread on dishes or bowls. Use salt and pepper to season the chicken salad and serve on the cress.

Nutrition:
- Calories: 368
- Protein: 37 g
- Fat: 14 g
- Carbohydrates: 22 g
- Added Sugar: 17 g
- Fibbers: 2 g

215. Cucumber Salad

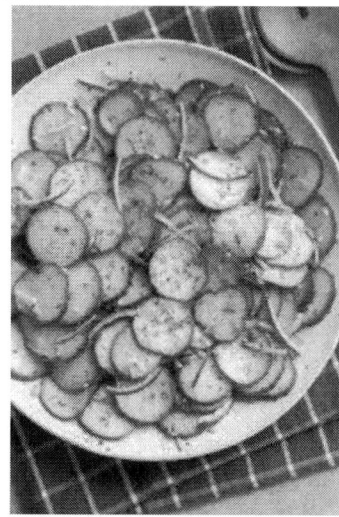

Preparation Time: 5 minutes
Cooking Time: 5 minutes
Servings: 4
Ingredients:
- 1 tbsp. dried dill
- 1 onion
- ¼ cup water
- 1 cup vinegar
- 3 cucumbers
- ¾ cup white sugar

Directions:
1. In a bowl add all ingredients and mix well
2. Serve with dressing

Nutrition:
- Calories: 49
- Fat: 0.1 g
- Sodium (Na): 341 mg
- Potassium (K): 171 mg
- Protein: 0.8 g
- Carbs: 11 g
- Phosphorus: 24 mg

216. Thai Cucumber Salad

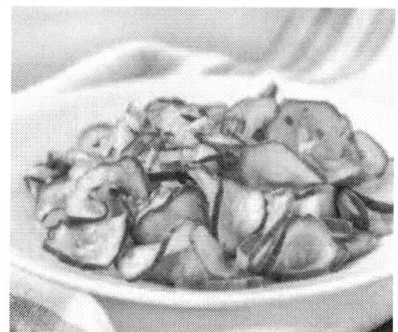

Preparation Time: 5 minutes
Cooking Time: 5 minutes
Servings: 2
Ingredients:
- ¼ cup chopped peanuts
- ¼ cup white sugar
- ½ cup cilantro
- ¼ cup rice wine vinegar
- 3 cucumbers
- 2 jalapeno peppers

Directions:
1. In a bowl, add all ingredients and mix well
2. Serve with dressing

Nutrition:
- Calories: 20
- Fat: 0 g
- Sodium (Na): 85 mg
- Carbs: 5 g
- Protein: 1 g
- Potassium (K): 190.4 mg
- Phosphorus: 46.8 mg

217. Broccoli-Cauliflower Salad

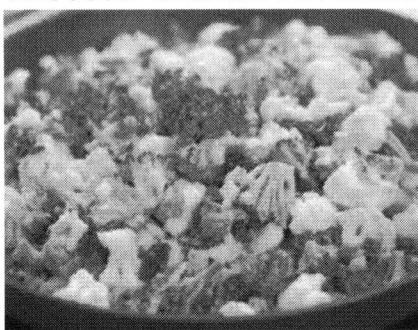

Preparation Time: 5 minutes
Cooking Time: 5 minutes
Servings: 4
Ingredients:
- 1 tbsp. wine vinegar
- 1 cup cauliflower florets
- ¼ cup white sugar
- 2 cups hard-cooked eggs
- 5 slices bacon
- 1 cup broccoli florets
- 1 cup cheddar cheese
- 1 cup mayonnaise

Directions:
1. In a bowl, add all ingredients and mix well
2. Serve with dressing

Nutrition:
- Calories: 89.8
- Fat: 4.5 g
- Sodium (Na): 51.2 mg
- Potassium (K) 257.6 mg
- Carbs: 11.5 g
- Protein: 3.0 g
- Phosphorus: 47 mg

218. Macaroni Salad

Preparation Time: 5 minutes
Cooking Time: 5 minutes
Servings: 4
Ingredients:
- ¼ tsp. celery seed
- 2 hard-boiled eggs
- 2 cups salad dressing
- 1 onion
- 2 tsps. white vinegar
- 2 stalks celery
- 2 cups cooked macaroni
- 1 red bell pepper
- 2 tbsps. mustard

Directions:
1. In a bowl, add all ingredients and mix well
2. Serve with dressing

Nutrition:
- Calories: 360
- Fat: 21 g
- Sodium (Na): 400 mg
- Carbs: 36 g
- Protein: 6 g
- Potassium: (K) 68 mg
- Phosphorus: 36 mg

CHAPTER 10:

Soup, Salad, Snacks & Light Meals Recipes

219. Cinnamon Apple Chips
Preparation Time: 5 minutes
Cooking Time: 2 to 3 hours
Servings: 4
Ingredients:
- 4 apples
- 1 teaspoon ground cinnamon

Directions:
1. Preheat the oven to 200°F. Line a baking sheet with parchment paper.
2. Core the apples and cut into ⅛-inch slices.
3. In a medium bowl, toss the apple slices with the cinnamon. Spread the apples in a single layer on the prepared baking sheet.
4. Cook for 2 to 3 hours, until the apples are dry. They will still be soft while hot but will crisp once completely cooled.
5. Store in an airtight container for up to four days.

Cooking Tip: If you don't have parchment paper, use cooking spray to prevent sticking.

Nutrition:
- Calories: 96 Total Fat: 0 g
- Saturated Fat: 0 g
- Cholesterol: 0 mg
- Carbohydrates: 26 g
- Fiber: 5 g Protein: 1 g
- Phosphorus: 0 mg
- Potassium: 198 mg
- Sodium: 2 mg

220. Roasted Red Pepper Hummus
Preparation Time: 10 minutes
Cooking Time: 10 minutes
Servings: 28
Ingredients:
- 1 red bell pepper
- 1 (15-ounce) can chickpeas, drained and rinsed
- Juice of 1 lemon
- 2 tablespoons tahini
- 2 garlic cloves
- 2 tablespoons extra-virgin olive oil

Directions:
1. Change an oven rack to the highest position. Heat the broiler to high.
2. Core the pepper and cut it into three or four large pieces. Arrange them on a baking sheet, skin-side up.
3. Broil the peppers for 5 to 10 minutes, until the skins are charred.
4. Cover with plastic wrap and let them steam for 10 to 15 minutes, until cool enough to handle.
5. Peel the skin off the peppers, and place the peppers in a blender.
6. Add the chickpeas, lemon juice, tahini, garlic, and olive oil.
7. Process until smooth, adding up to 1 tablespoon of water to adjust consistency as desired.

Substitution Tip: This hummus can also be made without the red pepper if desired. To do this, simply follow Step 5. This will cut the potassium to 59 mg per serving.

Nutrition:
- Total Fat: 6 g
- Saturated Fat: 1 g
- Cholesterol: 0 mg
- Carbohydrates: 10 g
- Fiber: 3 g
- Protein: 3 g
- Phosphorus: 58 mg
- Potassium: 91 mg
- Sodium: 72 mg

221. Thai-Style Eggplant Dip

Preparation Time: 10 minutes
Cooking Time: 30 minutes
Servings: 4
Ingredients:
- 1 pound Thai eggplant (or Japanese or Chinese eggplant)
- 2 tablespoons rice vinegar
- 2 teaspoons sugar
- 1 teaspoon low-sodium soy sauce
- 1 jalapeño pepper
- 2 garlic cloves
- ¼ cup chopped basil
- Cut vegetables for serving

Directions:
1. Preheat the oven to 475°F
2. Pierce the eggplant in several places with a skewer or knife. Place on a rimmed baking sheet and cook until soft, about 30 minutes.
3. Let cool, cut in half, and scoop out the flesh of the eggplant into a blender.
4. Add the rice vinegar, sugar, soy sauce, jalapeño, garlic, and basil to the blender. Process until smooth. Serve with cut vegetables
5. Lower sodium tip: If you need to lower your sodium further, omit the soy sauce to lower the sodium to 3mg.

Nutrition:
- Calories: 40
- Total Fat: 0g
- Saturated Fat: 0 g
- Cholesterol: 0 mg
- Carbohydrates: 10 g
- Fiber: 4 g
- Protein: 2 g
- Phosphorus: 34 mg
- Potassium: 284 mg
- Sodium: 47 mg

222. Collard Salad Rolls with Peanut Dipping Sauce

Preparation Time: 10 minutes
Cooking Time: 10 minutes
Servings: 4
Ingredients:
For the dipping sauce:
- ¼ cup peanut butter
- 2 tablespoons honey
- Juice of 1 lime
- ¼ teaspoon red chili flakes

For the salad rolls:
- 4 ounces' extra-firm tofu
- 1 bunch collard greens
- 1 cup thinly sliced purple cabbage
- 1 cup bean sprouts
- 2 carrots, cut into matchsticks
- ½ cup cilantro leaves and stems

Directions:
To make the dipping sauce:
1. In a blender, combine the peanut butter, honey, lime juice, chili

flakes, and process until smooth. Put 1 to 2 tablespoons of water as desired for consistency.

To make the salad rolls:
1. Using paper towels, press the excess moisture from the tofu. Cut into ½-inch-thick matchsticks.
2. Remove any tough stems from the collard greens and set aside.
3. Arrange all of the ingredients within reach. Cup one collard green leaf in your hand, and add a couple of pieces of the tofu and a small amount each of the cabbage, bean sprouts, and carrots. Top with a couple of cilantro sprigs, and roll into a cylinder. Place each roll, seam-side down, on a serving platter while you assemble the rest of the rolls. Serve with the dipping sauce.

Substitution Tip: To lower the potassium, omit the cabbage and use only 1 carrot, which will drop the potassium to 208 mg.

Nutrition:
- Calories: 174
- Total Fat: 9 g
- Saturated Fat: 2 g
- Cholesterol: 0 mg
- Carbohydrates: 20 g
- Fiber: 5 g
- Protein: 8 g
- Phosphorus: 56 mg
- Potassium: 284 mg
- Sodium: 42 mg

223. Simple Roasted Broccoli

Preparation Time: 5 minutes
Cooking Time: 20 minutes
Servings: 6
Ingredients:
- 2 small heads broccoli, cut into florets
- 1 tablespoon extra-virgin olive oil
- 3 garlic cloves, minced

Directions:
1. Preheat the oven to 425°F.
2. Toss the broccoli with the olive oil and garlic.
3. Arrange in a single layer on a baking sheet.
4. Roast for 10 minutes, then flip the broccoli and roast an additional 10 minutes. Serve.

Cooking Tip: Roasted broccoli makes for great leftovers—throw them in a quick salad for added flavor and bulk. To save leftovers, refrigerate in an airtight container for three to five days.

Nutrition:
- Calories: 38 Total Fat: 2 g
- Saturated Fat: 0 g
- Cholesterol: 0 mg
- Carbohydrates: 4 g
- Fiber: 1 g
- Protein: 1 g
- Phosphorus: 32 mg
- Potassium: 150 mg
- Sodium: 15 mg

224. Roasted Mint Carrots

Preparation Time: 20 minutes
Cooking Time: 5 minutes
Servings: 6
Ingredients:
- 1 pound carrots, trimmed
- 1 tablespoon extra-virgin olive oil

- Freshly ground black pepper
- ¼ cup thinly sliced mint

Directions:
1. Preheat the oven to 425°F.
2. Assemble the carrots in a single layer on a rimmed baking sheet. Drizzle with the olive oil, and shake the carrots on the sheet to coat. Season with pepper.
3. Cook for 20 minutes, or until tender and browned, stirring twice while cooking. Sprinkle with the mint and serve.

Substitution Tip: To lower the potassium in this dish, use 8 ounces of carrots and 8 ounces of turnips cut into cubes. This will cut the potassium to 193 mg.

Nutrition:
- Calories: 51
- Total Fat: 2 g
- Saturated Fat: 0 g
- Cholesterol: 0 mg
- Carbohydrates: 7 g
- Fiber: 2 g
- Protein: 1 g
- Phosphorus: 26 mg
- Potassium: 242 mg
- Sodium: 52 mg

225. Roasted Root Vegetables

Preparation Time: 10 minutes
Cooking Time: 25 minutes
Servings: 6
Ingredients:
- 1 cup chopped turnips
- 1 cup chopped rutabaga
- 1 cup chopped parsnips
- 1 tablespoon extra-virgin olive oil
- 1 teaspoon fresh chopped rosemary
- Freshly ground black pepper

Directions:
1. Preheat the oven to 420°F.
2. Toss the turnips, rutabaga, and parsnips with olive oil and rosemary.
3. Assemble in a single layer on a baking sheet, and season with pepper.
4. Roast until the vegetables are tender and browned, 20 to 25 minutes, stirring once.

Nutrition:
- Calories: 52
- Total Fat: 2 g
- Saturated Fat: 0 g
- Cholesterol: 0 mg
- Carbohydrates: 7 g
- Fiber: 2 g
- Protein: 1 g
- Phosphorus: 35 mg
- Potassium: 205 mg
- Sodium: 22 mg

226. Vegetable Couscous

Preparation Time: 10 minutes
Cooking Time: 51 minutes
Servings: 6
Ingredients:
- 1 tablespoon extra-virgin olive oil
- ½ sweet onion, diced
- 1 carrot, diced
- 1 celery stalk, diced
- ½ cup diced red or yellow bell pepper
- 1 small zucchini, diced
- 1 cup couscous
- 1½ cups Simple Chicken Broth or low-sodium store-bought chicken stock
- ½ teaspoon garlic powder
- Freshly ground black pepper

Directions:
1. Place the onion, carrot, celery, bell pepper, and cook, occasionally stirring until the vegetables are just becoming tender, about 5 to 7 minutes.
2. Add the zucchini, couscous, broth, and garlic powder.
3. Stir to blend and bring to a boil.
4. Cover and remove from the heat. Let stand for 5 to 8 minutes. Fluff with a fork, season with pepper and serve.

Nutrition:
- Calories: 154
- Total Fat: 3 g
- Saturated Fat: 1 g
- Cholesterol: 0 mg
- Carbohydrates: 27 g
- Fiber: 2 g
- Protein: 5 g
- Phosphorus: 83 mg
- Potassium: 197 mg
- Sodium: 36 mg

227. Garlic Cauliflower Rice
Preparation Time: 10 minutes
Cooking Time: 5 minutes
Servings: 8
Ingredients:
- 1 medium head cauliflower
- 1 tablespoon extra-virgin olive oil
- 4 garlic cloves, minced
- Freshly ground black pepper

Directions:
1. Using a sharp knife, remove the core of the cauliflower, and separate the cauliflower into florets.
2. In a food processor, pulse the florets until they are the size of rice, being careful not to overprocess them to the point of becoming mushy.
3. In a large skillet over medium heat, heat the olive oil. Add the garlic, and stir until just fragrant.
4. Add the cauliflower, stirring to coat. Add 1 tablespoon of water to the pan, cover, and reduce the heat to low. Steam for 7 to 10 minutes, until the cauliflower is tender. Season with pepper and serve.

Nutrition:
- Calories: 37
- Total Fat: 2 g
- Saturated Fat: 0 g
- Cholesterol: 0 mg
- Carbohydrates: 4 g
- Fiber: 2 g
- Protein: 2 g
- Phosphorus: 35 mg
- Potassium: 226 mg
- Sodium: 22 mg

228. Creamy Broccoli Soup
Preparation Time: 10 minutes
Cooking Time: 15 minutes
Servings: 4
Ingredients:
- 1 teaspoon extra-virgin olive oil
- ½ sweet onion, roughly chopped
- 2 cups chopped broccoli
- 4 cups low-sodium vegetable broth
- Freshly ground black pepper
- 1 cup Homemade Rice Milk or unsweetened store-bought rice milk
- ¼ cup grated Parmesan cheese

Directions:
1. Heat the olive oil. Add the onion and cook for 3 to 5 minutes, until it begins

to soften. Add the broccoli and broth, and season with pepper.
2. Bring to a boil, reduce the heat, and simmer open for 10 minutes, until the broccoli is just tender but still bright green.
3. Transfer the soup mixture to a blender. Add the rice milk, and process until smooth. Return to the saucepan, stir in the Parmesan cheese, and serve.

Nutrition:
- Calories: 88
- Total Fat: 3 g
- Saturated Fat: 1 g
- Cholesterol: 6 mg
- Carbohydrates: 12 g
- Fiber: 3 g
- Protein: 4 g
- Phosphorus: 87 mg
- Potassium: 201 mg
- Sodium: 281 mg

229. Curried Carrot and Beet Soup

Preparation Time: 10 minutes
Cooking Time: 50 minutes
Servings: 4
Ingredients:
- 1 large red beet
- 5 carrots, chopped
- 1 tablespoon curry powder
- 3 cups homemade rice milk or unsweetened store-bought rice milk
- Freshly ground black pepper
- Yogurt, for serving

Directions:
1. Preheat the oven to 400°F.
2. Wrap the beet in aluminum foil and roast for 45 minutes, until the vegetable is tender when pierced with a fork. Remove from the oven and let cool.
3. Add the carrots and cover with water. Bring to a boil, reduce the heat, cover, and simmer for 10 minutes until tender.
4. Transfer the carrots and beet to a food processor, and process until smooth. Add the curry powder and rice milk. Season with pepper. Serve topped with a dollop of yogurt.

Substitution Tip: Carrots are high in potassium. If you need to reduce your potassium further, use 2 carrots instead of 5. The soup will be a little thinner but still have a carrot flavor and just 322 mg of potassium.

Nutrition:
- Calories: 112
- Total Fat: 1 g
- Saturated Fat: 0 g
- Cholesterol: 0 mg
- Carbohydrates: 24 g
- Fiber: 7 g
- Protein: 3 g
- Phosphorus: 57 mg
- Potassium: 468 mg
- Sodium: 129 mg

230. Golden Beet Soup

Preparation Time: 10 minutes
Cooking Time: 35 minutes
Servings: 4
Ingredients:
- 3 tablespoons unsalted butter
- 4 golden beets, cut into ½-inch cubes
- ½ sweet onion, chopped
- 1-inch piece ginger, minced
- Zest and juice of 1 lemon
- 4 cups Simple Chicken Broth or low-sodium store-bought chicken stock

- Freshly ground black pepper
- ¼ cup pomegranate seeds, for servings
- ¼ cup crème fraîche, for servings (see Substitution tip)
- 10 sage leaves, for servings

Directions:
1. In a medium saucepan over medium heat, melt the butter.
2. Add the beets, onion, ginger, and lemon zest, and cover. Cook, occasionally stirring for 15 minutes. Add the broth, and continue to cook for 20 more minutes, until the beets are very tender.
3. In batches, transfer the soup to a blender and purée, or use an immersion blender.
4. Return the soup to the saucepan, and season with the pepper and lemon juice.
5. Serve topped with pomegranate seeds, crème fraîche, and sage leaves.

Substitution Tip: You can buy crème fraîche at many grocery stores or make your own. If you don't have crème fraîche, a dollop of whole-milk yogurt is a fine substitute.

Nutrition:
- Calories: 186
- Total Fat: 11 g
- Saturated Fat: 7 g
- Cholesterol: 26 mg
- Carbohydrates: 17 g
- Fiber: 3 g
- Protein: 7 g
- Phosphorus: 125 mg
- Potassium: 557 mg
- Sodium: 148 mg

231. Cauliflower and Chive Soup

Preparation Time: 10 minutes
Cooking Time: 20 minutes
Servings: 4
Ingredients:
- 2 tablespoons extra-virgin olive oil
- ½ sweet onion, chopped
- 2 garlic cloves, minced
- 2 cups Simple Chicken Broth or low-sodium store-bought chicken stock
- 1 cauliflower head, broken into florets
- Freshly ground black pepper
- 4 tablespoons (¼ cup) finely chopped chives

Directions:
1. Heat the olive oil.
2. Add the onion and cook, frequently stirring for 3 to 5 minutes, until it begins to soften. Add the garlic and stir until fragrant.
3. Add the broth and cauliflower, and bring to a boil. Reduce the heat and simmer until the cauliflower is tender for about 15 minutes.
4. Transfer the soup in batches to a blender or food processor and purée until smooth, or use an immersion blender.
5. Return the soup to the pot, and season with pepper before serving. Top each bowl with 1 tablespoon of chives.

Nutrition:
- Calories 132 Total Fat: 8 g
- Saturated Fat: 1 g
- Cholesterol: 0 mg
- Carbohydrates: 13 g Fiber: 3 g
- Protein: 6 g Phosphorus: 116 mg
- Potassium: 607 mg
- Sodium: 84 mg

232. Salad with Vinaigrette

Preparation Time: 25 minutes
Cooking Time: 0 minutes
Servings: 4
Ingredients:
For the vinaigrette:
- ½ cup olive oil
- 4 tbsps. balsamic vinegar
- 2 tbsps. chopped fresh oregano
- Pinch red pepper flakes
- Ground black pepper

For the salad:
- 4 cups shredded green leaf lettuce
- 1 carrot, shredded
- ¾ cup fresh green beans, cut into 1-inch pieces
- 3 large radishes, sliced thin

Directions:
1. To make the vinaigrette: put the vinaigrette ingredients in a bowl and whisk.
2. In a bowl, to make the salad, toss together the carrot, lettuce, green beans, and radishes.
3. Add the vinaigrette to the vegetables and toss to coat.
4. Arrange the salad on plates and serve.

Nutrition:
- Calories: 273
- Fat: 27 g
- Carbs: 7 g
- Phosphorus: 30 mg
- Potassium: 197 mg
- Sodium: 27 mg
- Protein: 1 g

233. Salad with Lemon Dressing

Preparation Time: 10 minutes
Cooking Time: 0 minutes
Servings: 4
Ingredients:
- ¼ cup heavy cream
- ¼ cup freshly squeezed lemon juice
- 2 tbsps. granulated sugar
- 2 tbsps. chopped fresh dill
- 2 tbsps. finely chopped scallion, green part only
- ¼ tsp. ground black pepper
- 1 English cucumber, thinly sliced
- 2 cups shredded green cabbage

Directions:
1. In a small bowl, stir together the lemon juice, cream, sugar, dill, scallion, and pepper until well blended.
2. In a large bowl, toss together the cucumber and cabbage.
3. Place the salad in the refrigerator and chill for 1 hour.
4. Stir before serving.

Nutrition:
- Calories: 99 Fat: 6 g
- Carbs: 13 g
- Phosphorus: 38 mg
- Potassium: 200 mg
- Sodium: 14 mg
- Protein: 2 g

234. Shrimp with Salsa

Preparation Time: 15 minutes
Cooking Time: 10 minutes
Servings: 4
Ingredients:
- 2 tbsp. olive oil

- 6 ounces large shrimp, peeled and deveined, tails left on
- 1 tsp. minced garlic
- ½ cup chopped English cucumber
- ½ cup chopped mango
- Zest of 1 lime
- Juice of 1 lime
- Ground black pepper
- Lime wedges for garnish

Directions:
1. Soak 4 wooden skewers in water for 30 minutes.
2. Preheat the barbecue to medium heat.
3. In a bowl, toss together the olive oil, shrimp, and garlic.
4. Line the shrimp onto the skewers, about 4 shrimp per skewer.
5. In a bowl, stir together the mango, cucumber, lime zest, and lime juice, and season the salsa lightly with pepper. Set aside.
6. Grill the shrimp for 10 minutes, turning once or until the shrimp is opaque and cooked through.
7. Season the shrimp lightly with pepper.
8. Serve the shrimp on the cucumber salsa with lime wedges on the side.

Nutrition:
- Calories: 120
- Fat: 8 g
- Carbs: 4 g
- Phosphorus: 91 mg
- Potassium: 129 mg
- Sodium: 60 mg
- Protein: 9 g

235. Cauliflower Soup

Preparation Time: 15 minutes
Cooking Time: 10 minutes
Servings: 4
Ingredients:
- 1 tsp unsalted butter.
- 1 small sweet onion, chopped
- 2 tsps. minced garlic
- Small head cauliflower1, cut into small florets
- 2 tsps. curry powder
- Water to cover the cauliflower
- ½ cup light sour cream
- 3 tbsps. chopped fresh cilantro

Directions:
1. Beat the butter over medium-high heat and sauté the onion-garlic for about 3 minutes or until softened.
2. Add the cauliflower, water, and curry powder.
3. Bring the soup to a simmer, then decrease the heat to low and simmer for 20 minutes or until the cauliflower is tender.
4. Puree the soup until creamy and smooth with a hand mixer.
5. Transfer the soup back into a saucepan and stir in the sour cream and cilantro.
6. Heat the soup on medium heat for 5 minutes or until warmed through.

Nutrition:
- Calories: 33 Fat: 2 g
- Carbs: 4 g
- Phosphorus: 30 mg
- Potassium: 167 mg
- Sodium: 22 mg
- Protein: 1 g

236. Cabbage Stew

Preparation Time: 20 minutes
Cooking Time: 35 minutes
Servings: 6
Ingredients:

- 1 tsp Unsalted butter
- ½ Large sweet onion, chopped
- 1 tsp Minced garlic
- 6 cups shredded green cabbage
- 3 Celery stalks chopped with leafy tops
- 1 Scallion, both green and white parts, chopped
- 2 tbsps. Chopped fresh parsley
- 2 tbsps. Freshly squeezed lemon juice
- 1 tbsp Chopped fresh thyme
- 1 tsp Chopped savory
- 1 tsp Chopped fresh oregano
- Water
- 1 cup fresh green beans, cut into 1-inch pieces
- Ground black pepper

Directions:

1. Melt the butter in a pot.
2. Sauté the onion and garlic in the melted butter for 3 minutes, or until the vegetables are softened.
3. Add the celery, cabbage, scallion, parsley, lemon juice, thyme, savory, and oregano to the pot, add enough water to cover the vegetables by 4 inches.
4. Bring the soup to a boil. Reduce the heat to low and simmer the soup for 25 minutes or until the vegetables are tender.
5. Season with pepper.

Nutrition:

- Calories: 33
- Fat: 1 g
- Carbs: 6 g
- Phosphorus: 29 mg
- Potassium: 187 mg
- Sodium: 20 mg
- Protein: 1 g

237. Eggplant and Red Pepper Soup

Preparation Time: 20 minutes
Cooking Time: 40 minutes
Servings: 6
Ingredients:

- 1 small sweet onion, cut into quarters
- 2 small red bell peppers, halved
- 2 cups cubed eggplant
- 2 cloves Garlic, crushed
- 1 tbsp. Olive oil
- 1 cup Chicken stock
- Water
- ¼ cup chopped fresh basil
- Ground black pepper

Directions:

1. Preheat the oven to 350F.
2. Put the onions, red peppers, eggplant, and garlic in a baking dish.
3. Drizzle the vegetables with the olive oil.
4. Roast the vegetables for 30 minutes or until they are slightly charred and soft.
5. Cool the vegetables slightly and remove the skin from the peppers.
6. Puree the vegetables with a hand mixer (with the chicken stock).
7. Transfer the soup to a medium pot and add enough water to reach the desired thickness.

8. Heat the soup to a simmer and add the basil.
9. Season with pepper and serve.

Nutrition:
- Calories: 61
- Fat: 2 g
- Carbs: 9 g
- Phosphorus: 33 mg
- Potassium: 198 mg
- Sodium: 98 mg
- Protein: 2 g

238. Kale Chips
Preparation Time: 20 minutes
Cooking Time: 25 minutes
Servings: 6
Ingredients:
- 2 cups Kale
- 2 tsp Olive oil
- ¼ tsp Chili powder
- Pinch cayenne pepper

Directions:
1. Preheat the oven to 300F.
2. Line 2 baking sheets with parchment paper set aside.
3. Remove the stems from the kale and tear the leaves into 2-inch pieces.
4. Wash the kale and dry it completely.
5. Handover the kale to a large bowl and drizzle with olive oil.
6. Use your hands to toss the kale with oil, taking care to coat each leaf evenly.
7. Season the kale with chili powder and cayenne pepper and toss to combine thoroughly.
8. Spread the seasoned kale in a single layer on each baking sheet. Do not overlap the leaves.
9. Bake the kale, rotating the pans once, for 20 to 25 minutes until it is crisp and dry.
10. Take out the oven trays and allow the chips to cool on the trays for 5 minutes.
11. Serve.

Nutrition:
- Calories: 24
- Fat: 2 g
- Carbs: 2 g
- Phosphorus: 21 mg
- Potassium: 111 mg
- Sodium: 13 mg
- Protein: 1 g

239. Tortilla Chips
Preparation Time: 15 minutes
Cooking Time: 10 minutes
Servings: 6
Ingredients:
- 2 tsps Granulated sugar –.
- ½ tsp. Ground cinnamon –
- Pinch ground nutmeg
- 3 (6-inch) flour tortillas
- Cooking spray

Directions:
1. Preheat the oven to 350F.
2. Line a baking sheet with parchment paper.
3. Mix the sugar, cinnamon, and nutmeg.
4. Lay the tortillas on a clean work surface and spray both sides of each lightly with cooking spray.
5. Sprinkle the cinnamon sugar evenly over both sides of each tortilla.

6. Cut the tortillas into 16 wedges each and place them on the baking sheet.
7. Bake the tortilla wedges, turning once, for about 10 minutes or until crisp.
8. Cool the chips and serve.

Nutrition:
- Calories: 51
- Fat: 1 g
- Carbs: 9 g
- Phosphorus: 29 mg
- Potassium: 24 mg
- Sodium: 103 mg
- Protein: 1 g

240. Corn Bread
Preparation Time: 10 minutes
Cooking Time: 20 minutes
Servings: 10
Ingredients:
- Cooking spray for greasing the baking dish
- 1 ¼ cups Yellow cornmeal
- ¾ cup All-purpose flour
- 1 tbsp Baking soda substitute
- ½ cup Granulated sugar
- 2 Eggs
- 1 cup Unsweetened, unfortified rice milk
- 2 tbsps Olive oil

Directions:
1. Preheat the oven to 425F.
2. Lightly spray an 8-by-8-inch baking dish with cooking spray. Set aside.
3. In a medium bowl, stir together the cornmeal, flour, baking soda substitute, and sugar.
4. In a small bowl, whisk together the eggs, rice milk, and olive oil until blended.
5. Place the wet ingredients into the dry ingredients and stir until well combined.
6. Pour the batter into the baking dish and bake for 20 minutes or until golden and cooked through.
7. Serve warm.

Nutrition:
- Calories: 198
- Fat: 5 g
- Carbs: 34 g
- Phosphorus: 88 mg
- Potassium: 94 mg
- Sodium: 25 mg
- Protein: 4 g

241. Vegetable Rolls
Preparation Time: 30 minutes
Cooking Time: 0 minutes
Servings: 8
Ingredients:
- ½ cup Finely shredded red cabbage
- ½ cup Grated carrot
- ¼ cup Julienne red bell pepper
- ¼ cup Julienned scallion, both green and white parts
- ¼ cup Chopped cilantro
- 1 tbsp Olive oil.
- ¼ tsp ground cumin
- ¼ tsp freshly ground black pepper
- 1 English cucumber sliced very thin strips

Directions:
1. In a bowl, toss together the black pepper, cumin, olive oil, cilantro, scallion, red pepper, carrot, and cabbage. Mix well.
2. Evenly divide the vegetable filling among the cucumber strips,

placing the filling close to one end of the strip.
3. Roll up the cucumber strips around the filling and secure with a wooden pick.
4. Repeat with each cucumber strip.

Nutrition:
- Calories: 26
- Fat: 2 g
- Carbs: 3 g
- Phosphorus: 14 mg
- Potassium: 95 mg
- Sodium: 7 mg
- Protein: 0 g

242. Frittata with Penne
Preparation Time: 15 minutes
Cooking Time: 30 minutes
Servings: 4
Ingredients:
- 6 Egg whites-
- ¼ cup Rice milk
- 1 tbsp Chopped fresh parsley
- 1 tsp Chopped fresh thyme.
- 1 tsp Chopped fresh chives
- Ground black pepper
- 2 tsps Olive oil
- ¼ Small sweet onion, chopped
- 1 tsp Minced garlic
- ½ cup Boiled and chopped red bell pepper
- 2 cups Cooked penne

Directions:
1. Preheat the oven to 350F.
2. Whisk together the egg whites, rice milk, parsley, thyme, chives, and pepper.
3. Heat the oil in a skillet.
4. Sauté the onion, garlic, red pepper for 4 minutes or until they are softened.
5. Add the cooked penne to the skillet.
6. Transfer the egg mixture over the pasta and shake the pan to coat the pasta.
7. Leave the skillet on the heat for 1 minute to set the bottom of the frittata
8. Bake the frittata for 25 minutes or until it is set and golden brown.
9. Serve.

Nutrition:
- Calories: 170
- Fat: 3 g
- Carbs: 25 g
- Phosphorus: 62 mg
- Potassium: 144 mg
- Sodium: 90 mg
- Protein: 10 g

243. Tofu Stir-Fry
Preparation Time: 20 minutes
Cooking Time: 20 minutes
Servings: 4
Ingredients:
For the tofu:
- 1 tbsp. Lemon juice
- 1 tsp Minced garlic
- 1 tsp Grated fresh ginger
- Pinch red pepper flakes
- 5 ounces Extra-firm tofu, pressed well and cubed

For the stir-fry:
- 1 tbsp Olive oil
- ½ cup Cauliflower florets
- ½ cup Thinly sliced carrots
- ½ cup Julienned red pepper

- ½ cup Fresh green beans
- 2 cups Cooked white rice

Directions:
1. Mix the lemon juice, garlic, ginger, and red pepper flakes.
2. Add the tofu and toss to coat.
3. Put the bowl in the refrigerator and soak for 2 hours.
4. To make the stir-fry, heat the oil in a skillet.
5. Sauté the tofu for 8 minutes or until it is lightly browned and heated through.
6. Add the carrots and cauliflower and sauté for 5 minutes. Stirring and tossing constantly.
7. Add the red pepper and green beans, sauté for 3 minutes more.
8. Serve over white rice.

Nutrition:
- Calories: 190
- Fat: 6 g
- Carbs: 30 g
- Phosphorus: 90 mg
- Potassium: 199 mg
- Sodium: 22 mg
- Protein: 6 g

244. Cauliflower Patties
Preparation Time: 5 minutes
Cooking Time: 8 minutes
Servings: 4
Ingredients:
- 2 Eggs
- 2 Egg whites
- ½, Onion, diced
- 2 cups Cauliflower, frozen
- 2 tbsps All-purpose white flour
- 1 tsp Black pepper
- 1 tbsp. Coconut oil

- 1 tsp Curry powder
- 1 tbsp Fresh cilantro

Directions:
1. Soak vegetables in warm water before cooking.
2. Steam cauliflower over a pan of boiling water for 10 minutes.
3. Blend eggs and onion in a food processor before adding cooked cauliflower, spices, cilantro, flour, and pepper, and blast in the processor for 30 seconds.
4. Heat a skillet on high heat and add oil.
5. Enjoy with a salad.

Nutrition:
- Calories: 227
- Fat: 12 g
- Carbs: 15 g
- Phosphorus: 193 mg
- Potassium: 513 mg
- Sodium: 158 mg
- Protein: 13 g

245. Turnip Chips
Preparation Time: 5 minutes
Cooking Time: 50 minutes
Servings: 2
Ingredients:
- 2 Turnips, peeled and sliced
- 1 tbsp Extra virgin olive oil
- 1 Onion chopped
- 1 clove minced garlic
- 1 tsp Black pepper
- 1 tsp Oregano
- 1 tsp Paprika

Directions:
1. Preheat oven to 375F. Grease a baking tray with olive oil.
2. Add turnip slices in a thin layer.

3. Dust over herbs and spices with an extra drizzle of olive oil.
4. Bake 40 minutes. Turning once.

Nutrition:
- Calories: 136
- Fat: 14 g
- Carbs: 30 g
- Phosphorus: 50 mg
- Potassium: 356 mg
- Sodium: 71 mg

246. Chicken and Mandarin Salad
Preparation Time: 40 minutes
Cooking Time: 30 minutes
Servings: 3
Ingredients:
- 1 ½ cup Chicken
- ½ cup Celery
- ½ cup Green pepper
- ¼ cup Onion, finely sliced
- ¼ cup Light mayonnaise
- ½ tsp. freshly ground pepper

Directions:
1. Hurl chicken, celery, green pepper, and onion to blend. Include mayo and pepper. Blend delicately and serve.

Nutrition:
- Calories: 375 Fat: 15 g
- Fiber: 2 g Carbs: 14 g
- Protein: 28 g

247. Roasted Red Pepper Soup
Preparation Time: 30 minutes
Cooking Time: 35 minutes
Servings: 4
Ingredients:
- 4 cups low-sodium chicken broth
- 3 red peppers
- 2 medium onions
- 3 tbsp. lemon juice
- 1 tbsp. finely minced lemon zest
- A pinch of cayenne pepper
- ¼ tsp. cinnamon
- ½ cup finely minced fresh cilantro

Directions:
1. In a medium stockpot, consolidate each one of the fixings except for the cilantro and warmth to the point of boiling over excessive warm temperature. Diminish the warmth and stew, ordinarily secured, for around 30 minutes, till thickened. Cool marginally. Utilizing a hand blender or nourishment processor, puree the soup. Include the cilantro and tenderly heat.

Nutrition:
- Calories: 266 Fat: 8 g
- Fiber: 6 g
- Carbs: 6 g
- Protein 31 g

248. Leek and Carrot Soup
Preparation Time: 15 minutes
Cooking Time: 25 minutes
Servings: 4
Ingredients:
- 1 leek
- ¾ cup diced and boiled carrots
- 1 garlic clove
- 1 tbsp oil
- Crushed pepper to taste
- 3 cups low sodium chicken stock
- Chopped parsley for garnish
- 1 bay leaf
- ¼ tsp ground cumin

Directions:
1. Trim off and take away a portion of the coarse inexperienced portions of the leek. At that factor, reduce daintily and flush altogether in water. Channel properly. Warmth the oil in an extensively based pot. Include the leek and garlic, and sear over low warmth for two-3 minutes, till sensitive. Include the inventory, inlet leaf, cumin, and pepper.
2. Heat the mixture to the point of boiling, mixing constantly. Include carrots and stew for 13 minutes. Modify the flavoring, eliminate the inlet leaf, and serve sprinkled with slashed parsley. To make a pureed soup, manner the soup in a blender or nourishment processor till smooth. Come again to the pan. Include ½ field milk. Bring to bubble and stew for 4 mins.

Nutrition:
- Calories: 325
- Fat: 9 g
- Fiber: 5 g
- Carbs: 16 g
- Protein: 29 g

249. Creamy Vinaigrette
Preparation Time: 15 minutes
Cooking Time: 25 minutes
Servings: 4
Ingredients:
- 2 tbsp. cider vinegar
- 2 tbsp. lime or lemon juice
- 1 garlic clove, minced
- 1 tsp. Dijon mustard
- 1 tsp. ground cumin
- ½ cup sour cream
- 2 tbsp. olive oil
- ¼ tsp. black pepper

Directions:
1. Consolidate all fixings and blend well. Fill serving of mixed greens carafe. Chill.

Nutrition:
- Calories: 188
- Fat: 15 g
- Fiber: 8 g
- Carbs: 35 g
- Protein: 25 g

250. Chicken and Pasta Salad
Preparation Time: 30 minutes
Cooking Time: 25 minutes
Servings: 6
Ingredients:
Chicken Pasta Salad:
- 6 oz. cooked chicken
- 3 cups pasta, spiral, cooked
- ½ green pepper, minced
- 1 ½ tbsp. onion
- ½ cup celery

Garlic Mustard Vinaigrette:
- 2 tbsp. cider Vinegar
- 2 tsp mustard, prepared
- ½ tsp. white sugar
- 1 garlic clove, Minced
- 1/3 cup water
- 1/3 cup olive oil
- 2 tsp. parmesan cheese, grated
- ½ tsp. ground pepper

Directions:
1. Combine all the chicken pasta salad ingredients.
2. In a little bowl, combine vinegar, mustard, sugar, garlic, and water

slowly race in oil. Mix in Parmesan. Season with pepper. Join 1/3 measure of dressing with chicken pasta salad and chill.

Nutrition:
- Calories: 233
- Fat: 12 g
- Fiber: 6 g
- Carbs: 25 g
- Protein: 23 g

251. Herbed Soup with Black Beans

Preparation Time: 10 minutes
Cooking Time: 10 minutes
Servings: 4
Ingredients:
- 2 tbsp tomato paste
- 1/3 cup Poblano pepper, charred, peeled, seeded and chopped
- 2 cups vegetable stock
- ¼ tsp cumin
- ½ tsp paprika
- ½ tsp dried oregano
- 2 tsp fresh garlic, minced
- 1 cup onion, small diced
- 1 tbsp extra-virgin olive oil
- 1 15-oz can black beans, drained and rinsed

Directions:
1. On medium fire, place a soup pot and heat oil. Add onion and sauté until translucent and soft, around 4-5 minutes. Add garlic, cook for 2 minutes.
2. Add the rest of the ingredients and bring to a simmer. Once simmering, turn off the fire and transfer to a blender. Puree ingredients until smooth.

Nutrition:
- Calories 98
- Fat: 21 g
- Fiber: 10 g
- Carbs: 20 g
- Protein: 19 g

252. Creamy Pumpkin Soup

Preparation Time: 10 minutes
Cooking Time: 20 minutes
Servings: 4
Ingredients:
- 1 onion, chopped
- 1 slice of bacon
- 2 tsp ground ginger
- 1 tsp cinnamon
- 1 cup applesauce
- 3 ½ cups low sodium chicken broth
- 1 29-oz can pumpkin
- Pepper to taste
- ½ cup light sour cream

Directions:
1. On medium-high fire, place a soup pot and add bacon once hot. Sauté until crispy, around 4 minutes. Discard bacon fat before continuing to cook. Add ginger, applesauce, chicken broth, and pumpkin. Lightly season with pepper. Bring to a simmer and cook for 11 minutes. Taste and adjust seasoning. Turn off fire, stir in sour cream and mix well.

Nutrition:
- Calories: 220 Fat: 8 g
- Fiber: 10 g
- Carbs: 36 g
- Protein: 10 g

253. Lemony Lentil Salad with Salmon

Preparation Time: 10 minutes
Cooking Time: 0 minutes
Servings: 3
Ingredients:
- ¼ tsp salt
- ½ cup chopped red onion
- 1 cup diced seedless cucumber
- 1 medium red bell pepper, diced
- 1/3 cup extra virgin olive oil
- 1/3 cup fresh dill, chopped
- 1/3 cup lemon juice
- 2 15oz cans of lentils
- 2 7oz cans of salmon, drained and flaked
- 2 tsp Dijon mustard
- Pepper to taste

Directions:
1. In a bowl, mix lemon juice, mustard, dill, salt, and pepper. Gradually add the oil, bell pepper, onion, cucumber, salmon flakes, and lentils. Toss to coat evenly.

Nutrition:
- Calories: 450
- Fat: 22 g
- Fiber: 10 g
- Carbs: 62 g
- Protein: 55 g

254. Spaghetti Squash & Yellow Bell-Pepper Soup

Preparation Time: 10 minutes
Cooking Time: 45 minutes
Servings: 4
Ingredients:
- 2 diced yellow bell peppers
- 2 chopped large garlic cloves
- 1 peeled and cubed spaghetti squash
- 1 quartered and sliced onion
- 1 tbsp. dried thyme
- 1 tbsp. coconut oil
- 1 tsp. curry powder
- 4 cups water

Directions:
1. Heat the oil in a large pan over medium-high heat before sweating the onions and garlic for 3-4 minutes.
2. Sprinkle over the curry powder.
3. Add the stock and bring to a boil over a high heat before adding the squash, pepper, and thyme.
4. Turn down the heat, cover, and allow to simmer for 25-30 minutes.
5. Continue to simmer until squash is soft if needed.
6. Allow cooling before blitzing in a blender/food processor until smooth.
7. Serve!

Nutrition:
- Calories: 103
- Protein: 2 g
- Carbs: 17 g
- Fat: 4 g
- Sodium (Na): 32 mg
- Potassium (K): 365 mg
- Phosphorus: 50 mg

255. Red Pepper & Brie Soup

Preparation Time: 10 minutes
Cooking Time: 35 minutes
Servings: 4
Ingredients:

- 1 tsp. paprika
- 1 tsp. cumin
- 1 chopped red onion
- 2 chopped garlic cloves
- ¼ cup crumbled brie
- 2 tbsps. extra virgin olive oil
- 4 chopped red bell peppers
- 4 cups water

Directions:

1. Heat the oil in a pot over medium heat.
2. Sweat the onions and peppers for 5 minutes.
3. Add the garlic cloves, cumin, and paprika and sauté for 3-4 minutes.
4. Add the water and allow to boil before turning the heat down to simmer for 30 minutes.
5. Remove from the heat and allow to cool slightly.
6. Put the mixture in a food processor and blend until smooth.
7. Pour into serving bowls and add the crumbled brie to the top with a little black pepper.
8. Enjoy!

Nutrition:

- Calories: 152
- Protein: 3 g
- Carbs: 8 g
- Fat: 11 g
- Sodium (Na): 66 mg
- Potassium (K): 270 mg
- Phosphorus: 207 mg

256. Turkey & Lemon-Grass Soup

Preparation Time: 5 minutes
Cooking Time: 40 minutes
Servings: 4
Ingredients:

- 1 fresh lime
- ¼ cup fresh basil leaves
- 1 tbsp. cilantro
- 1 cup chestnuts
- 1 tbsp. coconut oil
- 1 thumb-size minced ginger piece
- 2 chopped scallions
- 1 finely chopped green chili
- 4oz. skinless and sliced turkey breasts
- 1 minced garlic clove, minced
- ½ finely sliced stick lemon-grass
- 1 chopped white onion, chopped
- 4 cups water

Directions:

1. Crush the lemon-grass, cilantro, chili, 1 tbsp oil, and basil leaves in a blender or pestle and mortar to form a paste.
2. Heat a large pan/wok with 1 tbsp olive oil on high heat.
3. Sauté the onions, garlic, and ginger until soft.
4. Add the turkey and brown each side for 4-5 minutes.
5. Add the broth and stir.
6. Now add the paste and stir.
7. Next, add the chestnuts, turn down the heat slightly, and simmer for 25-30 minutes or until the turkey is thoroughly cooked through.

8. Serve hot with the green onion sprinkled over the top.

Nutrition:
- Calories: 123
- Protein: 10 g
- Carbs: 12 g
- Fat: 3 g
- Sodium (Na): 501 mg
- Potassium (K): 151 mg
- Phosphorus: 110 mg

257. Paprika Pork Soup

Preparation Time: 5 minutes
Cooking Time: 35 minutes
Servings: 2
Ingredients:
- 4 oz. sliced pork loin
- 1 tsp. black pepper
- 2 minced garlic cloves
- 3 cups water
- 1 tbsp. extra-virgin olive oil
- 1 chopped onion
- 1 tbsp. paprika

Directions:
1. In a large pot, add the oil, chopped onion, and minced garlic.
2. Sauté for 5 minutes on low heat.
3. Add the pork slices to the onions and cook for 7-8 minutes or until browned.
4. Add the water to the pan and bring to a boil on high heat.
5. Season with pepper to serve.

Nutrition:
- Calories: 165 Protein: 13 g
- Carbs: 10 g Fat: 9 g
- Sodium (Na): 269 mg
- Potassium (K): 486 mg
- Phosphorus: 158 mg

258. Mediterranean Vegetable Soup

Preparation Time: 5 minutes
Cooking Time: 30 minutes
Servings: 4
Ingredients:
- 1 tbsp. oregano
- 2 minced garlic cloves
- 1 tsp. black pepper
- 1 diced zucchini
- 1 cup diced eggplant
- 4 cups water
- 1 diced red pepper
- 1 tbsp. extra-virgin olive oil
- 1 diced red onion

Directions:
1. Soak the vegetables in warm water before use.
2. In a large pot, add the oil, chopped onion, and minced garlic.
3. Sweat for 5 minutes on low heat.
4. Add the other vegetables to the onions and cook for 7-8 minutes.
5. Add the stock to the pan and bring to a boil on high heat.
6. Stir in the herbs, reduce the heat, and simmer for a further 20 minutes or until thoroughly cooked through.
7. Season with pepper to serve.

Nutrition:
- Calories: 152
- Protein: 1 g
- Carbs: 6 g
- Fat: 3 g
- Sodium (Na): 3 mg
- Potassium (K): 229 mg
- Phosphorus: 45 mg

259. Tofu Soup

Preparation Time: 5 minutes
Cooking Time: 10 minutes
Servings: 2
Ingredients:
- 1 tbsp. miso paste
- 1/8 cup cubed soft tofu
- 1 chopped green onion
- ¼ cup sliced Shiitake mushrooms
- 3 cups Renali stock
- 1 tbsp. soy sauce

Directions:
1. Take a saucepan, pour the stock into this pan and let it boil on high heat. Reduce heat to medium and let this stock simmer. Add mushrooms to this stock and cook for almost 3 minutes.
2. Take a bowl and mix soy sauce (reduced salt) and miso paste together in this bowl. Add this mixture and tofu to stock. Simmer for nearly 5 minutes and serve with chopped green onion.

Nutrition:
- Calories: 129
- Fat 7.8 g
- Sodium (Na): 484 mg
- Potassium (K): 435 mg
- Protein: 11 g
- Carbs: 5.5 g
- Phosphorus :73.2 mg

260. Onion Soup

Preparation Time: 15 minutes
Cooking Time: 45 minutes
Servings: 6
Ingredients:
- 2 tbsps. chicken stock
- 1 cup chopped shiitake mushrooms
- 1 tbsp. minced chives
- 3 tsps. beef bouillon
- 1 tsp. grated ginger root
- ½ chopped carrot
- 1 cup sliced Portobello mushrooms
- 1 chopped onion
- ½ chopped celery stalk
- 2 quarts' water
- ¼ tsp. minced garlic

Directions:
1. Take a saucepan and combine carrot, onion, celery, garlic, mushrooms (some mushrooms), and ginger in this pan. Add water, beef bouillon, and chicken stock to this pan. Put this pot on high heat and let it boil. Decrease flame to medium and cover this pan to cook for almost 45 minutes.
2. Put all remaining mushrooms in one separate pot. Once the boiling mixture is completely done, put one strainer over this new bowl with mushrooms and strain cooked soup in this pot over mushrooms. Discard solid-strained materials.
3. Serve delicious broth with yummy mushrooms in small bowls and sprinkle chives over each bowl.

Nutrition:
- Calories: 22 Fat 0 g
- Sodium (Na): 602.3 mg
- Potassium (K): 54.1 mg
- Carbs: 4.9 g Protein: 0.6 g
- Phosphorus: 15.8 mg

261. Steakhouse Soup

Preparation Time: 15 minutes
Cooking Time: 25 minutes
Servings: 4
Ingredients:
- 2 tbsps. soy sauce
- 2 boneless and cubed chicken breasts.
- ¼ lb. halved and trimmed snow peas
- 1 tbsp. minced ginger root
- 1 minced garlic clove
- 1 cup water
- 2 chopped green onions
- 3 cups chicken stock
- 1 chopped carrot
- 3 sliced mushrooms

Directions:
1. Take a pot and combine ginger, water, chicken stock, Soy sauce (reduced salt), and garlic in this pot. Let them boil on medium heat, mix in chicken pieces, and let them simmer on low heat for almost 15 minutes to tender chicken.
2. Stir in carrot and snow peas and simmer for almost 5 minutes. Add mushrooms to this blend and continue cooking to tender vegetables for nearly 3 minutes. Mix in the chopped onion and serve hot.

Nutrition:
- Calories: 319 Carbs: 14 g
- Fat 15 g
- Potassium (K): 225 mg
- Protein: 29 g
- Sodium (Na): 389 mg
- Phosphorous: 190 mg

262. Pear & Brie Salad

Preparation Time: 15 minutes
Cooking Time: 0 minutes
Servings: 4
Ingredients:
- 1 tbsp. olive oil
- 1 cup arugula
- ½ lemon
- ½ cup pears
- ¼ cucumber
- ¼ cup chopped brie

Directions:
1. Peel and dice the cucumber.
2. Dice the pear.
3. Wash the arugula.
4. Combine salad in a serving bowl and crumble the brie over the top.
5. Whisk the olive oil and lemon juice together.
6. Drizzle over the salad.
7. Season with a little black pepper to taste and serve immediately.

Nutrition:
- Calories: 54
- Protein: 1 g
- Carbs: 12 g
- Fat: 7 g
- Sodium (Na): 57 mg
- Potassium (K): 115 mg
- Phosphorus: 67 mg

263. Caesar Salad

Preparation Time: 5 minutes
Cooking Time: 5 minutes
Servings: 4
Ingredients:
- 1 head romaine lettuce
- ¼ cup mayonnaise
- 1 tbsp. lemon juice
- 4 anchovy fillets

- 1 tsp. Worcestershire sauce
- Black pepper
- 5 garlic cloves
- 4 tbsps. Parmesan cheese
- 1 tsp. mustard

Directions:
1. In a bowl, mix all ingredients and mix well
2. Serve with dressing

Nutrition:
- Calories: 44
- Fat: 2.1 g
- Sodium (Na): 83 mg
- Potassium (K): 216 mg
- Carbs: 4.3 g
- Protein: 3.2 g
- Phosphorus: 45.6 mg

CHAPTER 11:

Spice Blends and Seasoning

264. Creole Seasoning Mix

Preparation Time: 5 minutes
Cooking Time: 5 minutes
Servings: Makes ¼ cup [1 teaspoon = 1 serving.]
Ingredients:
- 1 tablespoon sweet paprika
- 1 tablespoon garlic powder
- 2 teaspoons onion powder
- 2 teaspoons dried oregano
- 1 teaspoon cayenne pepper
- 1 teaspoon ground thyme
- 1 teaspoon freshly ground black pepper

Directions:
1. In a small bowl, mix the paprika, garlic powder, onion powder, oregano, cayenne pepper, thyme, and black pepper until the ingredients are well combined.
2. Transfer the seasoning mixture to a small container with a lid.
3. Store in a cool, dry place for up to 6 months.

Nutrition:
- Calories: 7
- Fat: 0 g
- Carbohydrates: 2 g
- Phosphorus: 8 mg
- Potassium: 35 mg
- Sodium: 1 mg
- Protein: 0 g

265. Adobo Seasoning Mix

Preparation Time: 5 minutes
Cooking Time: 5 minutes
Servings: Makes 1¼ cups [1 teaspoon = 1 serving]
Ingredients:
- 4 tablespoons garlic powder
- 4 tablespoons onion powder
- 4 tablespoons ground cumin
- 3 tablespoons dried oregano
- 3 tablespoons freshly ground black pepper
- 2 tablespoons sweet paprika
- 2 tablespoons ground chili powder
- 1 tablespoon ground turmeric
- 1 tablespoon ground coriander

Directions:
1. In a small bowl, mix the garlic powder, onion powder, cumin, oregano, black pepper, paprika, chili powder, turmeric, and coriander until the ingredients are well combined.
2. Transfer the seasoning mixture to a small container with a lid and store in a cool, dry place for up to 6 months.

Nutrition:
- Calories: 8 Fat: 0 g
- Carbohydrates: 2 g Phosphorus: 9 mg
- Potassium: 38 mg
- Sodium: 12 mg Protein: 0 g

266. Lamb and Pork Seasoning

Preparation Time: 5 minutes
Cooking Time: 5 minutes
Servings: Makes ½ cup [1 teaspoon = 1 serving]
Ingredients:
- ¼ cup celery seed
- 2 tablespoons dried oregano
- 2 tablespoons onion powder
- 1 tablespoon dried thyme
- 1½ teaspoons garlic powder
- 1 teaspoon crushed bay leaf
- 1 teaspoon freshly ground black pepper
- 1 teaspoon ground allspice

Directions:
1. Put the celery seed, oregano, onion powder, thyme, garlic powder, bay leaf, pepper, and allspice in a blender and pulse a few times to combine.
2. Transfer the herb mixture to a small container with a lid.
3. Store in a cool, dry place for up to 6 months.

Nutrition:
- Calories: 8
- Fat: 0 g
- Carbohydrates: 1 g
- Phosphorus: 9 mg
- Potassium: 29 mg
- Sodium: 2 mg
- Protein: 0 g

267. Asian Seasoning

Preparation Time: 5 minutes
Cooking Time: 5 minutes
Servings: Makes ½ cup [1 teaspoon = 1 serving]
Ingredients:
- 2 tablespoons sesame seeds
- 2 tablespoons onion powder
- 2 tablespoons crushed star anise pods
- 2 tablespoons ground ginger
- 1 teaspoon ground allspice
- ½ teaspoon cardamom
- ½ teaspoon ground cloves

Directions:
1. In a small bowl, mix the sesame seeds, onion powder, star anise, ginger, allspice, cardamom, and cloves until well combined.
2. Transfer the spice mixture to a small container with a lid.
3. Store in a cool, dry place for up to 6 months.

Nutrition:
- Calories: 10
- Fat: 0 g
- Carbohydrates: 1 g
- Phosphorus: 11 mg
- Potassium: 24 mg ;
- Sodium: 5 mg ;
- Protein: 0 g

268. Onion Seasoning Blend

Preparation Time: 5 minutes
Cooking time: 5 minutes
Servings: Makes ½ cup [1 teaspoon = 1 serving]
Ingredients:
- 2 tablespoons onion powder
- 1 tablespoon dry mustard
- 2 teaspoons sweet paprika
- 2 teaspoons garlic powder
- 1 teaspoon dried thyme
- ½ teaspoon celery seeds
- ½ teaspoon freshly ground black pepper

Directions:
1. In a small bowl, mix the onion powder, mustard, paprika, garlic powder, thyme, celery seeds, and pepper until well combined.
2. Transfer the spice mixture to a small container with a lid.
3. Store in a cool, dry place for up to 6 months.

Nutrition:
- Calories: 5
- Fat: 0 g
- Carbohydrates: 1 g
- Phosphorus: 6 mg
- Potassium: 17 mg
- Sodium: 1 mg
- Protein: 1 g

269. Apple Pie Spice
Preparation time: 5 minutes
Cooking Time: 5 minutes
Servings: Makes ⅓ cup [1 teaspoon = 1 serving]

Ingredients:
- ¼ cup ground cinnamon
- 2 teaspoons ground nutmeg
- 2 teaspoons ground ginger
- 1 teaspoon allspice
- ½ teaspoon ground cloves

Directions:
1. In a small bowl, mix the cinnamon, nutmeg, ginger, allspice, and cloves until the ingredients are well combined.
2. Transfer the spice mixture to a small container with a lid.
3. Store in a cool, dry place for up to 6 months.

Nutrition:
- Calories: 6
- Fat: 0 g
- Carbohydrates: 1 g
- Phosphorus: 2 mg
- Potassium: 12 mg
- Sodium: 1 mg
- Protein: 0 g

270. Poultry Seasoning
Preparation Time: 5 minutes
Cooking Time: 5 minutes
Servings: Makes ½ cup [1 teaspoon = 1 serving]

Ingredients:
- 2 tablespoons ground thyme
- 2 tablespoons ground marjoram
- 1 tablespoon ground sage
- 1 tablespoon ground celery seed
- 1 teaspoon ground rosemary
- 1 teaspoon freshly ground black pepper

Directions:
1. In a small bowl, mix the thyme, marjoram, sage, celery seed, rosemary, and pepper until the ingredients are well combined.
2. Transfer the seasoning mixture to a small container with a lid.
3. Store in a cool, dry place for up to 6 months.

Nutrition:
- Calories: 3
- Fat: 0 g
- Carbohydrates: 0 g
- Phosphorus: 3 mg
- Potassium: 10 mg
- Sodium: 1 mg
- Protein: 0 g

271. Hot Curry Powder

Preparation Time: 5 minutes
Cooking Time: 5 minutes
Servings: Makes 1¼ cups [1 tablespoon = 1 serving]
Ingredients:
- ¼ cup ground cumin
- ¼ cup ground coriander
- 3 tablespoons turmeric
- 2 tablespoons sweet paprika
- 2 tablespoons ground mustard
- 1 tablespoon fennel powder
- ½ teaspoon green chili powder
- 2 teaspoons ground cardamom
- 1 teaspoon ground cinnamon
- ½ teaspoon ground cloves

Directions:
1. Put the cumin, coriander, turmeric, paprika, mustard, fennel powder, green chili powder, cardamom, cinnamon, and cloves into a blender, and pulse until the ingredients are ground and well combined.
2. Transfer the curry powder to a small container with a lid.
3. Store in a cool, dry place for up to 6 months.

Dialysis Modification: Omit the sweet paprika to reduce the amount of potassium. It will change the curry powder's color, but the other spices have a strong enough flavor to make up for the omission.

Nutrition:
- Calories: 19 Fat: 1 g
- Carbohydrates: 3 g
- Phosphorus: 24 mg
- Potassium: 93 mg
- Sodium: 5 mg
- Protein: 1 g

272. Cajun Seasoning

Preparation Time: 5 minutes
Cooking Time: 5 minutes
Servings: Makes 1¼ cups [1 teaspoon = 1 serving]
Ingredients:
- ½ cup sweet paprika
- ¼ cup garlic powder
- 3 tablespoons onion powder
- 3 tablespoons freshly ground black pepper
- 2 tablespoons dried oregano
- 1 tablespoon cayenne pepper
- 1 tablespoon dried thyme

Directions:
1. Put the paprika, garlic powder, onion powder, black pepper, oregano, cayenne pepper, thyme in a blender, and pulse until the ingredients are ground and well combined.
2. Transfer the seasoning mixture to a small container with a lid.
3. Store in a cool, dry place for up to 6 months.

Nutrition:
- Calories: 7 Fat: 0 g
- Carbohydrates: 2 g
- Phosphorus: 8 mg
- Potassium: 40 mg
- Sodium: 1 mg
- Protein: 0 g

273. Berbere spice mix

Preparation Time: 5 minutes
Cooking Time: 5 minutes
Servings: Makes ½ cup [1 teaspoon = 1 serving]
Ingredients:
- 1 tablespoon coriander seeds
- 1 teaspoon cumin seeds

- 1 teaspoon fenugreek seeds
- ¼ teaspoon black peppercorns
- ¼ teaspoon whole allspice berries
- 4 whole cloves
- 4 dried chilies, stemmed and seeded
- ¼ cup dried onion flakes
- 2 tablespoons ground cardamom
- 1 tablespoon sweet paprika
- 1 teaspoon ground ginger
- ½ teaspoon ground nutmeg
- ½ teaspoon ground cinnamon

Directions:
1. In a small skillet over medium heat, add the coriander, cumin, fenugreek, peppercorns, allspice, and cloves.
2. Lightly toast the spices, swirling the skillet constantly, for about 4 minutes or until the spices are fragrant.
3. Remove the skillet from the heat and let the spices cool for about 10 minutes.
4. Transfer the toasted spices to a blender with the chilies and onion, and grind until the mixture is finely ground.
5. Transfer the ground spice mixture to a small bowl and stir together the cardamom, paprika, ginger, nutmeg, and cinnamon until thoroughly combined.
6. Store the spice mixture in a small container with a lid for up to 6 months.

Nutrition:
- Calories: 8
- Fat: 0 g
- Carbohydrates: 2 g
- Phosphorus: 7 mg
- Potassium: 37 mg
- Sodium: 14 mg
- Protein: 0 g

CHAPTER 12:

Vegetables

274. Thai Tofu Broth
Preparation Time: 5 minutes
Cooking Time: 15 minutes
Servings: 4
Ingredients:
- 1 cup rice noodles
- ½ sliced onion
- 6 oz. drained, pressed, and cubed tofu
- ¼ cup sliced scallions
- ½ cup water
- ½ cup chestnuts
- ½ cup rice milk
- 1 tbsp. lime juice
- 1 tbsp. coconut oil
- ½ finely sliced chili
- 1 cup snow peas

Directions:
1. Heat the oil in a wok on high heat and then sauté the tofu until brown on each side.
2. Add the onion and sauté for 2-3 minutes.
3. Add the rice milk and water to the wok until bubbling.
4. Lower to medium heat and add the noodles, chili, and water chestnuts.
5. Allow to simmer for 10-15 minutes, and then add the sugar snap peas for 5 minutes.
6. Serve with a sprinkle of scallions.

Nutrition:
- Calories: 304
- Total Fat: 13 g
- Saturated Fat: 0 g
- Cholesterol: 0 mg
- Sodium: 36 mg
- Total Carbs: 38 g
- Fiber: 0 g
- Sugar: 0 g
- Protein: 9 g

275. Delicious Vegetarian Lasagna
Preparation Time: 10 minutes
Cooking Time: 1 hour
Servings: 4
Ingredients:
- 1 tsp. basil
- 1 tbsp. olive oil
- ½ sliced red pepper
- 3 lasagna sheets
- ½ diced red onion
- ¼ tsp. black pepper
- 1 cup rice milk
- 1 minced garlic clove
- 1 cup sliced eggplant
- ½ sliced zucchini
- ½ pack soft tofu
- 1 tsp. oregano

Directions:
1. Preheat oven to 325°F/Gas Mark 3.
2. Slice zucchini, eggplant, and pepper into vertical strips.
3. Add the rice milk and tofu to a food processor and blitz until smooth. Set aside.
4. Heat the oil in a skillet over medium heat and add the onions and garlic for 3-4 minutes or until soft.
5. Sprinkle in the herbs and pepper and allow to stir through for 5-6 minutes until hot.
6. Into a lasagna or suitable oven dish, layer 1 lasagna sheet, then 1/3 the eggplant, followed by 1/3 zucchini, then 1/3 pepper before pouring over 1/3 of white tofu sauce.
7. Repeat for the next 2 layers, finishing with the white sauce.
8. Add to the oven for 40-50 minutes or until veg is soft and easily be sliced into servings.

Nutrition:
- Calories: 235 Total Fat: 9 g
- Saturated Fat: 0 g
- Cholesterol: 0 mg
- Sodium: 35 mg
- Total Carbs: 10 g Fiber: 0 g
- Sugar: 0 g Protein: 5 g

276. Chili Tofu Noodles
Preparation Time: 5 minutes
Cooking Time: 15 minutes
Servings: 4
Ingredients:
- ½ diced red chili
- 2 cups rice noodles
- ½ juiced lime
- 6 oz. pressed and cubed silken firm tofu
- 1 tsp. grated fresh ginger
- 1 tbsp. coconut oil
- 1 cup green beans
- 1 minced garlic clove

Directions:
1. Steam the green beans for 10-12 minutes or according to package directions and drain.
2. Cook the noodles in a pot of boiling water for 10-15 minutes or according to package directions.
3. Meanwhile, heat a wok or skillet on high heat and add coconut oil.
4. Now add the tofu, chili flakes, garlic, and ginger and sauté for 5-10 minutes.
5. Drain the noodles and add to the wok along with the green beans and lime juice.
6. Toss to coat.
7. Serve hot!

Nutrition:
- Calories: 246
- Total Fat: 12 g
- Saturated Fat: 0 g
- Cholesterol: 0 mg
- Sodium: 25 mg
- Total Carbs: 28 g
- Fiber: 0 g
- Sugar: 0 g
- Protein: 10 g

277. Curried Cauliflower
Preparation Time: 5 minutes
Cooking Time: 20 minutes
Servings: 4
Ingredients:
- 1 tsp. turmeric
- 1 diced onion
- 1 tbsp. chopped fresh cilantro
- 1 tsp. cumin
- ½ diced chili
- ½ cup water
- 1 minced garlic clove
- 1 tbsp. coconut oil
- 1 tsp. garam masala
- 2 cups cauliflower florets

Directions:
1. Add the oil to a skillet on medium heat.
2. Sauté the onion and garlic for 5 minutes until soft.
3. Add the cumin, turmeric, and garam masala and stir to release the aromas.
4. Now add the chili to the pan along with the cauliflower.
5. Stir to coat.
6. Pour in the water and reduce the heat to a simmer for 15 minutes.
7. Garnish with cilantro to serve.

Nutrition:
- Calories: 108
- Total Fat: 7 g
- Saturated Fat: 0 g
- Cholesterol: 0 mg
- Sodium: 35 mg
- Total Carbs: 11 g
- Fiber: 0 g
- Sugar: 0 g
- Protein: 2 g

278. Chinese Tempeh Stir Fry
Preparation Time: 5 minutes
Cooking Time: 15 minutes
Servings: 2
Ingredients:
- 2 oz. sliced tempeh
- 1 cup cooked rice
- 1 minced garlic clove
- ½ cup green onions
- 1 tsp. minced fresh ginger
- 1 tbsp. coconut oil
- ½ cup corn

Directions:
1. Heat the oil in a skillet or wok on high heat and add the garlic and ginger.
2. Sauté for 1 minute.
3. Now add the tempeh and cook for 5-6 minutes before adding the corn for a further 10 minutes.
4. Now add the green onions and serve over rice.

Nutrition:
- Calories: 304 Total Fat: 4 g
- Saturated Fat: 0 g
- Cholesterol: 0 mg
- Sodium: 91 mg
- Total Carbs: 35 g Fiber: 0 g
- Sugar: 0 g Protein: 10 g

279. Egg White Frittata with Penne
Preparation Time: 15 minutes
Cooking Time: 30 minutes
Servings: 4
Ingredients:
- 6 Egg whites
- ¼ cup Rice milk
- 1 tbsp Chopped fresh parsley
- 1 tsp Chopped fresh thyme

- 1 tsp Chopped fresh chives
- Ground black pepper
- 2 tsp Olive oil
- ¼ Small sweet onion, chopped
- 1 tsp Minced garlic
- ½ cup Boiled and chopped red bell pepper
- 2 cups Cooked penne

Directions:
1. Preheat the oven to 350f.
2. In a bowl, whisk together the egg whites, rice milk, parsley, thyme, chives, and pepper.
3. Heat the oil in a skillet.
4. Sauté the onion, garlic, red pepper for 4 minutes or until they are softened.
5. Add the cooked penne to the skillet.
6. Pour the egg mixture over the pasta and shake the pan to coat the pasta.
7. Leave the skillet on the heat for 1 minute to set the frittata's bottom and then transfer the skillet to the oven.
8. Bake the frittata for 25 minutes, or until it is set and golden brown.
9. Serve.

Nutrition:
- Calories: 170 Total Fat: 3 g
- Saturated Fat: 0 g
- Cholesterol: 0 mg
- Sodium: 90 mg
- Total Carbs: 25 g
- Fiber: 0 g Sugar: 0 g
- Protein: 10 g

280. Vegetable Fried Rice
Preparation time: 20 minutes
Cooking time: 20 minutes
Servings: 6 servings
Ingredients:
- Olive oil – 1 tbsp.
- Sweet onion – ½, chopped
- Grated fresh gingcr – 1 tbsp.
- Minced garlic - 2 tsp
- Sliced carrots – 1 cup
- Chopped eggplant – ½ cup
- Peas – ½ cup
- Green beans – ½ cup, cut into 1-inch pieces
- Chopped fresh cilantro – 2 tbsp.
- Cooked rice – 3 cups

Directions:
1. Heat the olive oil in a skillet.
2. Sauté the ginger, onion, and garlic for 3 minutes or until softened.
3. Stir in carrot, eggplant, green beans, and peas and sauté for 3 minutes more.
4. Add cilantro and rice.
5. Sauté, constantly stirring, for about 10 minutes or until the rice is heated through.
6. Serve.

Nutrition:
- Calories: 189 Total Fat: 7 g
- Saturated Fat: 0 g
- Cholesterol: 0 mg
- Sodium: 13 mg
- Total Carbs: 28 g
- Fiber: 0 g Sugar: 0 g
- Protein: 6 g

281. Vegetable Biryani

Preparation Time: 20 minutes
Cooking Time: 10 minutes
Servings: 4
Ingredients:

- 2 tablespoons olive oil
- 1 onion, diced
- 4 garlic cloves, minced
- 1 tablespoon peeled and grated fresh ginger root
- 1 cup carrot, grated
- 2 cups chopped cauliflower
- 1 cup frozen baby peas, thawed and drained
- 2 teaspoons curry powder
- 1 cup low-sodium vegetable broth
- 3 cups frozen cooked rice

Directions:

Biryani is an Indian dish made of rice and vegetables that are spiced with curry powder. If you are new to curry powder, try several brands and add the one you like best. Curry powder can be mild or fiery hot, depending on the ingredients used in the blend. This recipe is simple to make and can be bulked up by stuffing the rice mixture into a pita.

1. In a large skillet, heat the olive oil over medium heat.
2. Add the onion, garlic, and ginger root and sauté, frequently stirring until tender-crisp, 2 minutes.
3. Add the carrot, cauliflower, peas, and curry powder and cook for 2 minutes longer.
4. Stir in the vegetable broth and bring to a simmer. Reduce the heat to low, partially cover the skillet, and simmer for 6 to 7 minutes or until the vegetables are tender.
5. Meanwhile, heat the rice as directed on the package.
6. Stir the rice into the vegetable mixture and serve.

Nutrition:

- Calories: 378 Total Fat: 16 g
- Saturated Fat: 2 g
- Cholesterol: 0 mg
- Sodium: 113 mg
- Total Carbs: 53 g Fiber: 7 g
- Sugar: 6 g Protein: 8 g

282. Couscous Burgers

Preparation Time: 20 minutes
Cooking Time: 10 minutes
Servings: 4
Ingredients:

- ½ cup chickpeas
- 2 tbsp. Chopped fresh cilantro
- Chopped fresh parsley
- 1 tbsp. Lemon juice
- 2 tsp Lemon zest
- 1 tsp Minced garlic
- 2 ½ cups Cooked couscous
- 2 Eggs, lightly beaten
- 2 tbsp. Olive oil

Directions:

1. Put the cilantro, chickpeas, parsley, lemon juice, lemon zest, and garlic in a food processor and pulse until a paste form.
2. Transfer the chickpea mixture to a bowl, and add the eggs and couscous. Mix well.
3. Chill the mixture in the refrigerator for 1 hour.
4. Form the couscous mixture into 4 patties.
5. Heat olive oil in a skillet.

6. Place the patties in the skillet, 2 at a time, gently pressing them down with the fork of a spatula.
7. Cook for 5 minutes or until golden, and flip the patties over.
8. Cook the other side for 5 minutes and transfer the cooked burgers to a plate covered with a paper towel.
9. Repeat with the remaining 2 burgers.

Nutrition:
- Calories: 242 Total Fat: 10 g
- Saturated Fat: 0 g
- Cholesterol: 0 mg
- Sodium: 43 mg Total Carbs: 29 g
- Fiber: 0 g Sugar: 0 g
- Protein: 9 g

283. Marinated Tofu Stir-Fry
Preparation Time: 20 minutes
Cooking Time: 20 minutes
Servings: 4
Ingredients:
For the tofu:
- 1 tbsp Lemon juice.
- 1 tsp Minced garlic
- 1 tsp Grated fresh ginger
- Pinch red pepper flakes
- 5 ounces Extra-firm tofu, pressed well and cubed

For the stir-fry:
- 1 tbsp Olive oil
- ½ cup Cauliflower florets
- ½ cup Thinly sliced carrots
- ½ cup Julienned red pepper
- ½ cup Fresh green beans
- 2 cups Cooked white rice

Directions:
1. In a bowl, mix the lemon juice, garlic, ginger, and red pepper flakes.
2. Add the tofu and toss to coat.
3. Place the bowl in the refrigerator and marinate for 2 hours.
4. To make the stir-fry, heat the oil in a skillet.
5. Sauté the tofu for 8 minutes or until it is lightly browned and heated through.
6. Add the carrots and cauliflower and sauté for 5 minutes. Constantly stirring and tossing.
7. Add the red pepper and green beans, sauté for 3 minutes more.
8. Serve over white rice.

Nutrition:
- Calories: 190
- Total Fat: 6 g
- Saturated Fat: 0 g
- Cholesterol: 0 mg
- Sodium: 22 mg
- Total Carbs: 30 g
- Fiber: 0 g
- Sugar: 0 g
- Protein: 6 g

284. Curried Veggie Stir-Fry

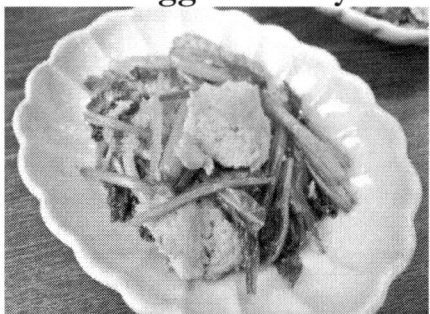

Preparation Time: 20 minutes
Cooking Time: 10 minutes
Servings: 6
Ingredients:
- 2 tablespoons of extra-virgin olive oil

- 1 onion, chopped
- 4 garlic cloves, minced
- 4 cups of frozen stir-fry vegetables
- 1 cup unsweetened full-fat coconut milk
- 1 cup of water
- 2 tablespoons of green curry paste

Directions:
1. In a wok or non-stick, heat the olive oil over medium-high heat. Stir-fry the onion and garlic for 2 to 3 minutes, until fragrant.
2. Add the frozen stir-fry vegetables and continue to cook for 3 to 4 minutes longer, or until the vegetables are hot.
3. Meanwhile, in a small bowl, combine coconut milk, water, and curry paste. Stir until the paste dissolves.
4. Add the broth mixture to the wok and cook for another 2 to 3 minutes, or until the sauce has reduced slightly and all the vegetables are crisp-tender.
5. Serve over couscous or hot cooked rice.

Nutrition:
- Calories: 293
- Total fat: 18 g
- Saturated fat: 10 g
- Sodium: 247 mg
- Phosphorus: 138 mg
- Potassium: 531 mg
- Carbohydrates: 28 g
- Fiber: 7 g
- Protein: 7 g
- Sugar: 4 g

285. Chilaquiles

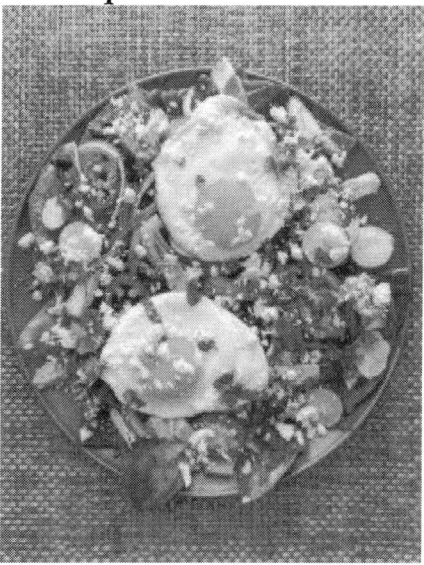

Preparation Time: 20 minutes
Cooking Time: 20 minutes
Servings: 4
Ingredients:
- 3 (8-inch) corn tortillas, cut into strips
- 2 tablespoons of extra-virgin olive oil
- 12 tomatillos, papery covering removed, chopped
- 3 tablespoons for freshly squeezed lime juice
- 1/8 teaspoon of salt
- 1/8 teaspoon of freshly ground black pepper
- 4 large egg whites
- 2 large eggs
- 2 tablespoons of water
- 1 cup of shredded pepper jack cheese

Directions:
1. In a dry nonstick skillet, toast the tortilla strips over medium heat until they are crisp, tossing the pan and

occasionally stirring. This should take 4 to 6 minutes. Remove the strips from the pan and set aside.
2. In the same skillet, heat the olive oil over medium heat and add the tomatillos, lime juice, salt, and pepper. Cook and frequently stir for about 8 to 10 minutes until the tomatillos break down and form a sauce. Transfer the sauce to a bowl and set aside.
3. In a small bowl, beat the egg whites, eggs, and water and add to the skillet. Cook the eggs for 3 to 4 minutes, occasionally stirring until they are set and cooked to 160°F.
4. Preheat the oven to 400°F.
5. Toss the tortilla strips in the tomatillo sauce and place in a casserole dish. Top with the scrambled eggs and cheese.
6. Bake for 10 to 15 minutes, or until the cheese starts to brown. Serve.

Nutrition:
- Calories: 312
- Total Fat: 20 g
- Saturated Fat: 8 g
- Sodium: 345 mg
- Phosphorus: 280 mg
- Potassium: 453 mg
- Carbohydrates: 19 g
- Fiber: 3 g
- Protein: 15 g
- Sugar: 5 g

286. Roasted Veggie Sandwiches

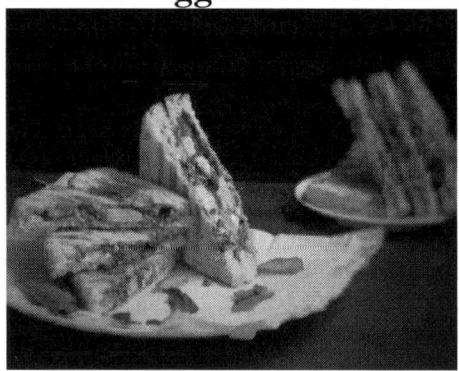

Preparation Time: 20 minutes
Cooking Time: 35 minutes
Servings: 6
Ingredients:
- 3 bell peppers, assorted colors, sliced
- 1 cup of sliced yellow summer squash - 1 red onion, sliced
- 2 tablespoons of extra-virgin olive oil - 2 tablespoons of balsamic vinegar
- ⅛ teaspoon of salt
- ⅛ teaspoon of freshly ground black pepper
- 3 large whole-wheat pita breads, halved

Directions:
1. Preheat the oven to 400°F.
2. Prepare a parchment paper and line it with a rimmed baking sheet.
3. Spread the bell peppers, squash, and onion on the prepared baking sheet. Sprinkle with the olive oil, vinegar, salt, and pepper.
4. Roast for 30 to 40 minutes, turning the vegetables with a spatula once during cooking until they are tender and light golden brown.

5. Pile the vegetables into the pieces of pita bread and serve.

Nutrition:
- Calories: 182
- Total Fat: 5 g
- Saturated Fat: 1 g
- Sodium: 234 mg
- Phosphorus: 106 mg
- Potassium: 289 mg
- Carbohydrates: 31 g
- Fiber: 4 g
- Protein: 5 g
- Sugar: 6 g

287. Pasta Fagioli

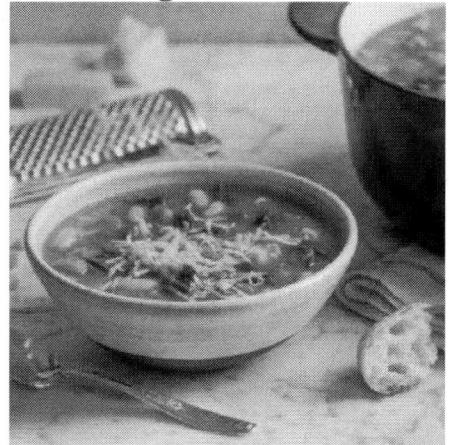

Preparation Time: 25 minutes
Cooking Time: 25 minutes
Servings: 6
Ingredients:
- 1 (15-ounce) can low-sodium great northern beans, drained and rinsed, divided
- 2 cups frozen peppers and onions, thawed, divided
- 5 cups low-sodium vegetable broth
- ⅛ teaspoon salt
- ⅛ teaspoon freshly ground black pepper
- 1 cup whole-grain orecchiette pasta
- 2 tablespoons extra-virgin olive oil
- ⅓ cup grated Parmesan cheese

Directions:
1. In a large saucepan, place the beans and cover with water. Bring to a boil over high heat and boil for 10 minutes. Drain the beans.
2. In a food processor or blender, combine ⅓ cup of beans and ⅓ cup of thawed peppers and onions. Process until smooth.
3. In the same saucepan, combine the pureed mixture, the remaining 1⅔ cups of peppers and onions, the remaining beans, the broth, and the salt and pepper, and bring to a simmer.
4. Add the pasta to the saucepan. Make sure to stir it and bring it to boil, reduce the heat to low, and simmer for 8 to 10 minutes, or until the pasta is tender.
5. Serve drizzled with olive oil and topped with Parmesan cheese.

Nutrition:
- Calories: 245
- Total Fat: 7 g
- Saturated Fat: 2 g
- Sodium: 269 mg
- Phosphorus: 188 mg
- Potassium: 592 mg
- Carbohydrates: 36 g
- Fiber: 7 g
- Protein: 12 g
- Sugar: 4 g

288. Roasted Peach Open-Face Sandwich

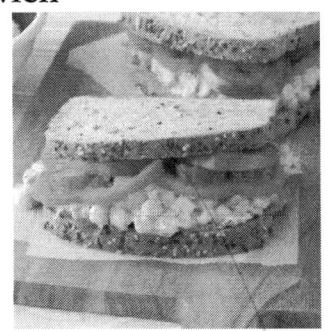

Preparation Time: 5 minutes
Cooking Time: 15 minutes
Servings: 4
Ingredients:
- 2 fresh peaches, peeled and sliced
- 1 tablespoon of extra-virgin olive oil
- 1 tablespoon of freshly squeezed lemon juice
- ⅛ teaspoon of salt
- ⅛ teaspoon of freshly ground black pepper
- 4 ounces of cream cheese, at room temperature
- 2 teaspoons of fresh thyme leaves
- 4 bread slices

Directions:
1. Preheat the oven to 400°F.
2. Arrange the peaches on a rimmed baking sheet. Brush them with olive oil on both sides.
3. Roast the peaches for 10 to 15 minutes, until they are lightly golden brown around the edges. Sprinkle with lemon juice, salt, and pepper.
4. In a small bowl, combine the cream cheese and thyme and mix well.
5. Toast the bread. Get the toasted bread and spread it with the cream cheese mixture. Top with the peaches and serve.

Nutrition:
- Calories: 250 Total Fat: 13 g
- Saturated Fat: 6 g
- Sodium: 376 mg
- Phosphorus: 163 mg
- Potassium: 260 mg
- Carbohydrates: 28 g
- Fiber: 3 g Protein: 6 g
- Sugar: 8 g

289. Spicy Corn and Rice Burritos

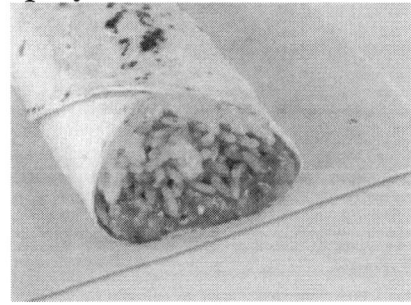

Preparation Time: 10 minutes
Cooking Time: 20 minutes
Servings: 4
Ingredients:
- 3 tablespoons of extra-virgin olive oil, divided
- 1 (10-ounce) package of frozen cooked rice
- 1½ cups of frozen yellow corn
- 1 tablespoon of chili powder
- 1 cup of shredded pepper jack cheese
- 4 large or 6 small corn tortillas

Directions:
1. Put the skillet in over medium heat and put 2 tablespoons of olive oil. Add the rice, corn, and chili powder and cook for 4 to 6 minutes, or until the ingredients are hot.

2. Transfer the ingredients from the pan into a medium bowl. Let cool for 15 minutes.
3. Stir the cheese into the rice mixture.
4. Heat the tortillas using the directions from the package to make them pliable. Fill the corn tortillas with the rice mixture, then roll them up.
5. At this point, you can serve them as is, or you can fry them first. Heat the remaining tablespoon of olive oil in a large skillet. Fry the burritos, seam-side down at first, turning once, until they are brown and crisp, about 4 to 6 minutes per side, then serve.

Nutrition:
- Calories: 386 Total Fat: 21 g
- Saturated Fat: 7 g Sodium: 510 mg
- Phosphorus: 304 mg
- Potassium: 282 mg
- Carbohydrates: 41 g Fiber: 4 g
- Protein: 11 g Sugar: 2 g

290. Crustless Cabbage Quiche

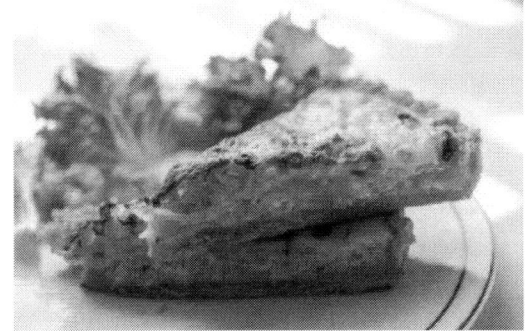

Preparation Time: 10 minutes
Cooking Time: 40 minutes
Servings: 6
Ingredients:
- Olive oil cooking spray
- 2 tablespoons of extra-virgin olive oil
- 3 cups of coleslaw blend with carrots
- 3 large eggs, beaten
- 3 large egg whites, beaten
- ½ cup of half-and-half
- 1 teaspoon of dried dill weed
- ⅛ teaspoon of salt
- ⅛ teaspoon of freshly ground black pepper
- 1 cup of grated Swiss cheese

Directions:
1. Preheat the oven to 350°F. Spray pie plate (9-inch) with cooking spray and set aside.
2. In a skillet, put oil and put it in medium heat. Add the coleslaw mix and cook for 4 to 6 minutes, stirring, until the cabbage is tender. Transfer the vegetables from the pan to a medium bowl to cool.
3. Meanwhile, in another medium bowl, combine the eggs and egg whites, half-and-half, dill, salt, and pepper, and beat to combine.
4. Stir the cabbage mixture into the egg mixture and pour into the prepared pie plate.
5. Sprinkle with the cheese.
6. Bake for 30 to 35 minutes, or until the mixture is puffed, set, and light golden brown. Let stand for 5 minutes, then slice to serve.

Nutrition:
- Calories: 203 Total Fat: 16 g
- Saturated Fat: 6 g Sodium: 321 mg
- Phosphorus: 169 mg
- Potassium: 155 mg
- Carbohydrates: 5 g
- Fiber: 1 g Protein: 11 g
- Sugar: 4 g

291. Vegetable Confetti Relish

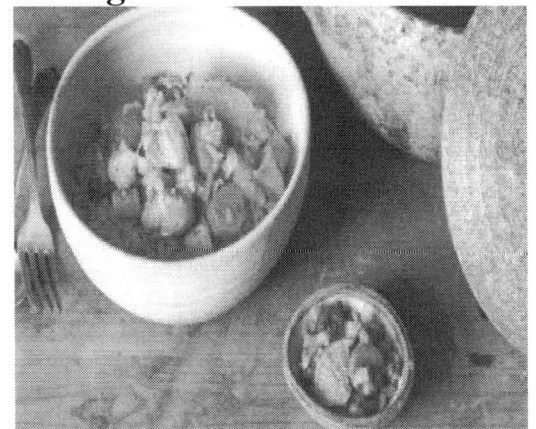

Preparation Time: 25 minutes
Cooking Time: 15 minutes
Servings: 1
Ingredients:
- ½ red bell pepper
- ½ green pepper, boiled and chopped
- 4 scallions, thinly sliced
- ½ tsp. of ground cumin
- 3 tbsp. of vegetable oil
- 1 ½ tbsp. of white wine vinegar
- Black pepper to taste

Directions:
1. Join all fixings and blend well.
2. Chill in the fridge.
3. You can include a large portion of slashed jalapeno pepper for an increasingly fiery blend

Nutrition:
- Calories: 230
- Fat: 25 g
- Fiber: 3 g
- Carbs: 24 g
- Protein: 43 g

292. Creamy Veggie Casserole

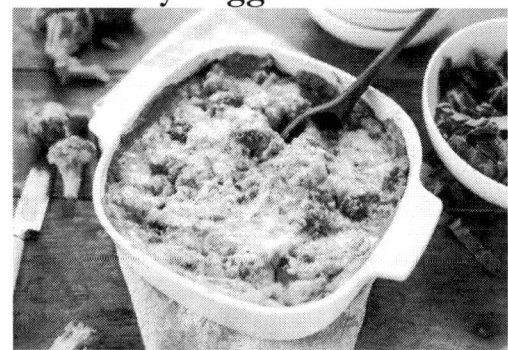

Preparation Time: 25 minutes
Cooking Time: 35 minutes
Servings: 4
Ingredients:
- ⅓ cup extra-virgin olive oil, divided
- 1 onion, chopped
- 2 tablespoons flour
- 3 cups low-sodium vegetable broth
- 3 cups frozen California blend vegetables
- 1 cup crushed crisp rice cereal

Directions:
1. Preheat the oven to 375°F.
2. Next is heat 2 tablespoons of olive oil in a large skillet over medium heat. Add the onion and cook for 3 to 4 minutes, stirring, until the onion is tender.
3. Add the flour and stir for 2 minutes.
4. Add the broth to the saucepan, stirring for 3 to 4 minutes, or until the sauce starts to thicken.
5. Add the vegetables to the saucepan. Simmer and cook until vegetables are tender (for six to eight minutes).
6. When the vegetables are done, pour the mixture into a 3-quart casserole dish.
7. Sprinkle the vegetables with the crushed cereal.

8. Bake for 20 to 25 minutes or until the cereal is golden brown and the filling is bubbling. Let cool for 5 minutes and serve.

Nutrition:
- Calories: 234 Total fat: 18 g
- Saturated fat: 3 g
- Sodium: 139 mg
- Phosphorus: 21 mg
- Potassium: 210 mg
- Carbohydrates: 16 g Fiber: 3 g
- Protein: 3 g Sugar: 5 g

293. Vegetable Green Curry

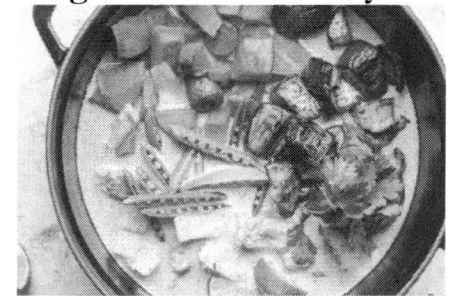

Preparation Time: 20 minutes
Cooking Time: 20 minutes
Servings: 6
Ingredients:
- 2 tablespoons extra-virgin olive oil
- 1 head broccoli, cut into florets
- 1 bunch asparagus, cut into 2-inch lengths
- 3 tablespoons water
- 2 tablespoons green curry paste
- 1 medium eggplant
- ⅛ teaspoon salt
- ⅛ teaspoon freshly ground black pepper
- ⅔ cup plain whole-milk yogurt

Directions:
1. Put olive oil in a large saucepan in a medium heat. Add the broccoli and stir-fry for 5 minutes. Add the asparagus and stir-fry for another 3 minutes.
2. Meanwhile, in a small bowl, combine the water with the green curry paste.
3. Add the eggplant, curry-water mixture, salt, and pepper. Stir-fry or until vegetables are all tender.
4. Add the yogurt. Heat through but avoid simmering. Serve.

Nutrition:
- Calories: 113 Total fat: 6 g
- Saturated fat: 1 g Sodium: 174 mg
- Phosphorus: 117 mg
- Potassium: 569 mg
- Carbohydrates: 13 g Fiber: 6 g
- Protein: 5 g Sugar: 7 g

294. Zucchini Bowl

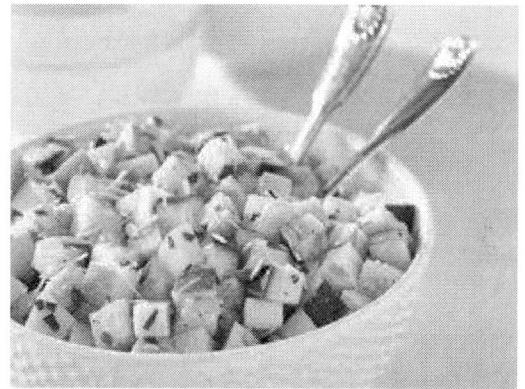

Preparation Time: 10 minutes
Cooking Time: 20 minutes
Servings: 4
Ingredients:
- 1 onion, chopped
- 3 zucchini, cut into medium chunks
- 2 tablespoons coconut milk
- 2 garlic cloves, minced
- 4 cups chicken stock
- 2 tablespoons coconut oil
- Pinch of salt

- Black pepper to taste

Directions:
1. Take a pot and place it over medium heat
2. Add oil and let it heat up
3. Add zucchini, garlic, onion, and stir
4. Cook for 5 minutes
5. Add stock, salt, pepper, and stir
6. Bring to a boil and lower down the heat
7. Simmer for 20 minutes.
8. Remove heat and add coconut milk
9. Use an immersion blender until smooth
10. Ladle into soup bowls and serve

Enjoy!

Nutrition:
- Calories: 160 Fat: 2 g
- Carbohydrates: 4 g Protein: 7 g

295. Nice Coconut Haddock

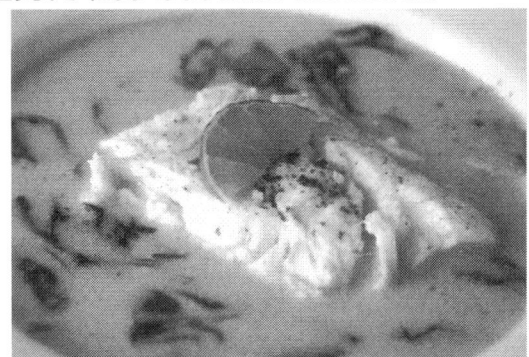

Preparation Time: 10 minutes
Cooking Time: 12 minutes
Servings: 3
Ingredients:
- 4 haddock fillets, 5 ounces each, boneless
- 2 tablespoons coconut oil, melted
- 1 cup coconut, shredded and unsweetened
- ¼ cup hazelnuts, ground
- Salt to taste

Directions:
1. Preheat your oven to 400 °F
2. Line a baking sheet with parchment paper
3. Keep it on the side
4. Pat fish fillets with a paper towel and season with salt
5. Take a bowl and stir in hazelnuts and shredded coconut
6. Drag fish fillets through the coconut mix until both sides are coated well
7. Transfer to a baking dish
8. Brush with coconut oil
9. Bake for about 12 minutes until flaky

Serve and enjoy!

Nutrition:
- Calories: 299
- Fat: 24 g
- Carbohydrates: 1 g
- Protein: 20 g

296. Vegetable Rice Casserole

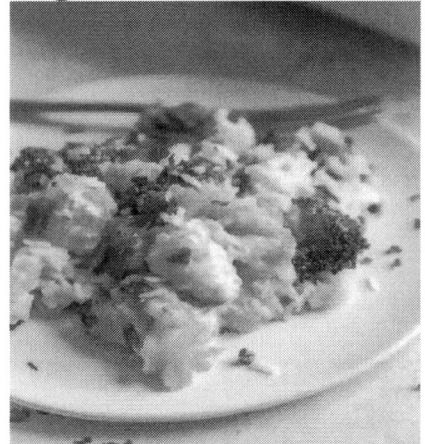

Preparation Time: 10 minutes
Cooking Time: 50 minutes
Servings: 4
Ingredients:
- 1 teaspoon of olive oil

- ½ small sweet onion, chopped
- ½ teaspoon of minced garlic
- ½ cup of chopped red bell pepper
- ¼ cup of grated carrot
- 1 cup of white basmati rice
- 2 cups of water
- ¼ cup of grated Parmesan cheese
- Freshly ground black pepper

Directions:
1. Preheat the oven to 350°f.
2. In a medium skillet over medium-high heat, heat the olive oil.
3. Add the onion and garlic, and sauté until softened, about 3 minutes.
4. Transfer the vegetables to a 9-by-9-inch baking dish, and stir in the rice and water.
5. Cover the dish and bake until the liquid is absorbed 35 to 40 minutes.
6. Sprinkle the cheese on top and bake an additional 5 minutes to melt.
7. Season the casserole with pepper, and serve.

Substitution tip: Not surprisingly, the cheesy topping on this casserole elevates it to a truly sublime experience. You can also try feta, Cheddar cheese, and goat cheese for different tastes and textures.

Nutrition:
- Calories: 224
- Total fat: 3 g
- Saturated fat: 1 g
- Cholesterol: 6 mg
- Sodium: 105 mg
- Carbohydrates: 41 g
- Fiber: 2 g
- Phosphorus: 118 mg
- Potassium: 176 mg
- Protein: 6 g
- Kidney Disease Stage 1

CHAPTER 13:

Smoothies and Drinks

297. Almonds & Blueberries Smoothie

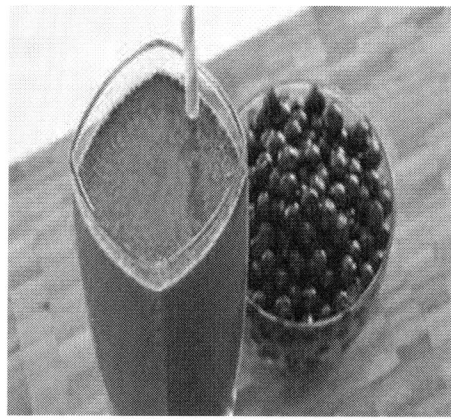

Preparation Time: 5 minutes
Cooking Time: 3 minutes
Servings: 2
Ingredients:

- ¼ cup ground almonds, unsalted
- 1 cup fresh blueberries
- Fresh juice of a 1 lemon
- 1 cup fresh Kale leaf
- ½ cup coconut water
- 1 cup water
- 2 tbsp. plain yogurt (optional)

Directions:
1. Dump all ingredients in your high-speed blender, and blend until your smoothie is smooth.
2. Pour the mixture into a chilled glass.
3. Serve and enjoy!

Nutrition:
- Calories: 110
- Carbohydrates: 8 g
- Proteins: 2 g
- Fat: 7 g
- Fiber: 2 g

298. Almonds and Zucchini Smoothie

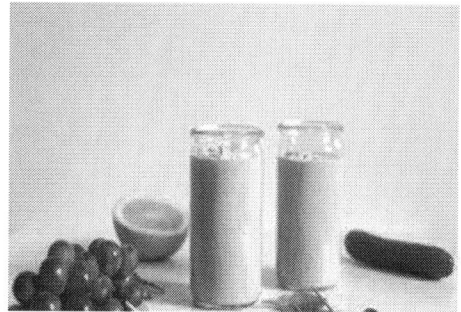

Preparation Time: 5 minutes
Cooking Time: 3 minutes
Servings: 2
Ingredients:

- 1 cup zucchini, cooked and mashed - unsalted
- 1 ½ cups almond milk
- 1 Tbsp. almond butter (plain, unsalted)
- 1 tsp pure almond extract
- 2 Tbsp. ground almonds or Macadamia almonds
- ½ cup water

- 1 cup Ice cubes crushed (optional, for serving)

Directions:
1. Dump all ingredients from the list above in your fast-speed blender; blend for 45 - 60 seconds or as you prefer.
2. Serve with crushed ice.

Nutrition:
- Calories: 322
- Carbohydrates: 6 g
- Proteins: 6 g
- Fat: 30 g
- Fiber: 3.5 g

299. Blueberries and Coconut Smoothie

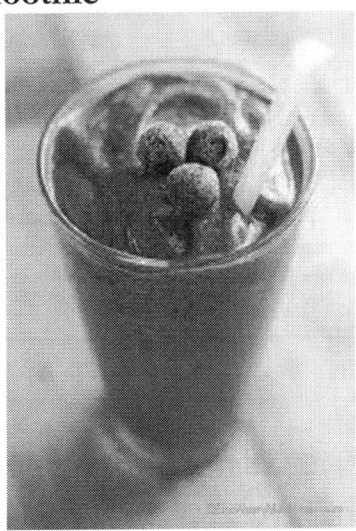

Preparation Time: 5 minutes
Cooking Time: 3 minutes
Servings: 5
Ingredients:
- 1 cup of frozen blueberries, unsweetened
- 1 cup Stevia or Erythritol sweetener
- 2 cups coconut milk
- 2 tbsp. shredded coconut (unsweetened)
- 3/4 cups of water

Directions:
1. Place all ingredients from the list in the food processor or your strong blender.
2. Blend for 45 - 60 seconds or to taste.
3. Ready to drink! Serve!

Nutrition:
- Calories: 190
- Carbohydrates: 8 g
- Proteins: 3 g
- Fat: 18 g
- Fiber: 2 g

300. Collard Greens and Cucumber Smoothie

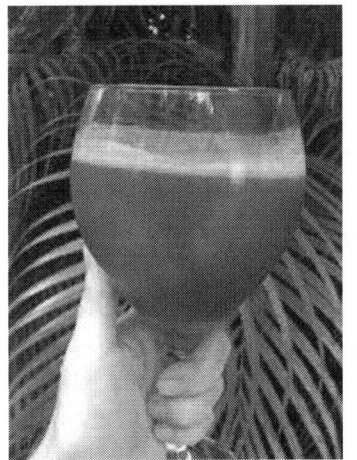

Preparation Time: 15 minutes
Cooking Time: 5 minutes
Servings: 2
Ingredients:
- 1 cup Collard greens
- A few fresh peppermint leaves
- 1 big cucumber
- 1 lime, freshly juiced

- 1 ½ cups of water
- 1 cup crushed ice
- ¼ cup of natural sweetener Erythritol or Stevia (optional)

Directions:
1. Rinse and clean your Collard greens from any dirt.
2. Place all the ingredients in a food processor or blender,
3. Blend until all the ingredients in your smoothie are mixed well.
4. Pour in a glass and drink. Enjoy!

Nutrition:
- Calories: 123
- Carbohydrates: 8 g
- Proteins: 4 g
- Fat: 11 g
- Fiber: 6 g

301. Creamy Dandelion Greens and Celery Smoothie

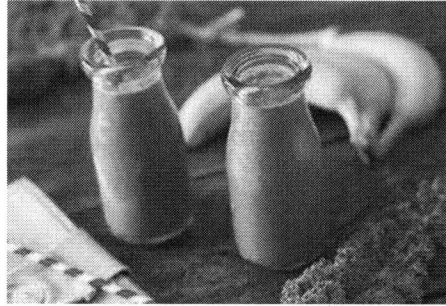

Preparation Time: 10 minutes
Cooking Time: 3 minutes
Servings: 2
Ingredients:
- 1 handful of raw dandelion greens
- 2 celery sticks
- 2 Tbsp. chia seeds
- 1 small piece of ginger, minced
- ½ cup almond milk

- ½ cup of water
- ½ cup plain yogurt

Directions:
1. Rinse and clean dandelion leaves from any dirt; add in a high-speed blender.
2. Clean the ginger; keep only the inner part and cut into small slices; add in a blender.
3. Add all remaining ingredients and blend until smooth.
4. Serve and enjoy!

Nutrition:
- Calories: 58
- Carbohydrates: 5 g
- Proteins: 3 g
- Fat: 6 g
- Fiber: 3 g

302. Dark Turnip Greens Smoothie

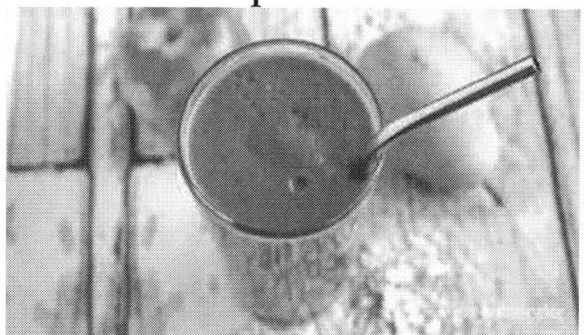

Preparation Time: 10 minutes
Cooking Time: 3 minutes
Servings: 2
Ingredients:
- 1 cup of raw turnip greens
- 1 ½ cup of almond milk
- 1 Tbsp. of almond butter
- ½ cup of water
- ½ tsp of cocoa powder, unsweetened

- 1 Tbsp. of dark chocolate chips
- ¼ tsp of cinnamon
- A pinch of salt
- ½ cup of crushed ice

Directions:
1. Rinse and clean turnip greens from any dirt.
2. Place the turnip greens in your blender along with all the other ingredients.
3. Blend it for 45 - 60 seconds or until done; smooth and creamy.
4. Serve with or without crushed ice.

Nutrition:
- Calories: 131
- Carbohydrates: 6 g
- Proteins: 4 g
- Fat: 10 g
- Fiber: 2.5 g

303. Butter Pecan and Coconut Smoothie

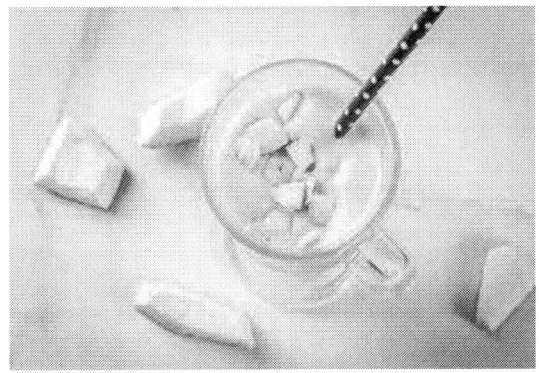

Preparation Time: 5 minutes
Cooking Time: 2 minutes
Servings: 2
Ingredients:
- 1 cup coconut milk
- 1 scoop Butter Pecan powdered creamer
- 2 tbsp. stevia granulated sweetener to taste
- ½ cup water
- 1 cup ice cubes crushed

Directions:
1. Place Ingredients from the list above in your high-speed blender.
2. Blend for 35 - 50 seconds or until all ingredients are combined well.
3. Add less or more crushed ice.
4. Drink and enjoy!

Nutrition:
- Calories: 268
- Carbohydrates: 7 g
- Proteins: 6 g
- Fat: 26 g
- Fiber: 1.5 g

304. Fresh Cucumber, Kale, and Raspberry Smoothie

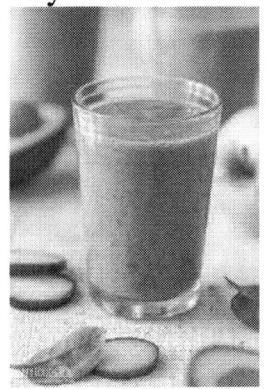

Preparation Time: 10 minutes
Cooking Time: 0 minutes
Servings: 3
Ingredients:
- 1 ½ cups of cucumber, peeled
- ½ cup raw kale leaves
- 1 ½ cups fresh raspberries

- 1 cup of almond milk
- 1 cup of water
- Ice cubes crushed (optional)
- 2 Tbsp. natural sweetener (Stevia, Erythritol...etc.)

Directions:
1. Place all ingredients from the list in a food processor or high-speed blender; blend for 35 - 40 seconds.
2. Serve into chilled glasses.
3. Add more natural sweeter if you like. Enjoy!

Nutrition:
- Calories: 70
- Carbohydrates: 8 g
- Proteins: 3 g
- Fat: 6 g
- Fiber: 5 g

305. Green Coconut Smoothie

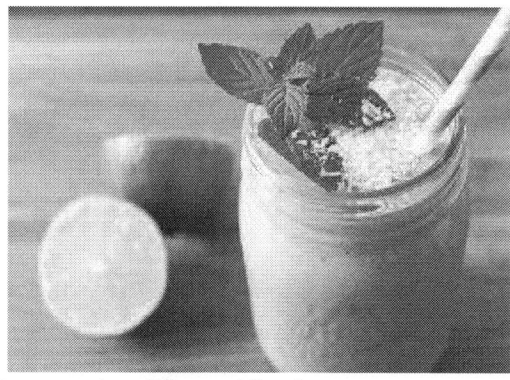

Preparation Time: 10 minutes
Cooking Time: 5 minutes
Servings: 2 servings
Ingredients:
- 1 ¼ cup coconut milk
- 2 Tbsp. chia seeds
- 1 cup of fresh kale leaves
- 1 scoop vanilla protein powder
- 1 cup ice cubes
- Granulated stevia sweetener (to taste; optional)
- ½ cup water

Directions:
1. Rinse and clean kale
2. Add all ingredients to your blender.
3. Blend until you get a nice smoothie.
4. Serve into chilled glass.

Nutrition:
- Calories: 179
- Carbohydrates: 5 g
- Proteins: 4 g
- Fat: 18 g
- Fiber: 2.5 g

306. Fresh Lettuce and Cucumber-Lemon Smoothie

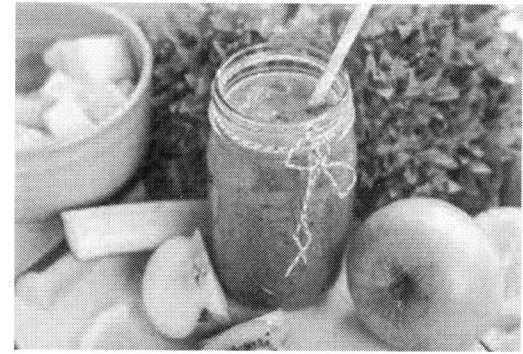

Preparation Time: 10 minutes
Cooking Time: 3 minutes
Servings: 2
Ingredients:
- 2 cups fresh lettuce leaves, chopped (any kind)
- 1 cup of cucumber
- 2 Tbsp. chia seeds
- 1 ½ cup water or coconut water
- ¼ cup stevia granulate sweetener (or to taste)

Directions:
1. Add all ingredients from the list above to the high-speed blender; blend until completely smooth.
2. Pour your smoothie into chilled glasses, and enjoy!

Nutrition:
- Calories: 51
- Carbohydrates: 4 g
- Proteins: 2 g
- Fat: 4 g
- Fiber: 3.5 g

307. Instant Coffee Smoothie

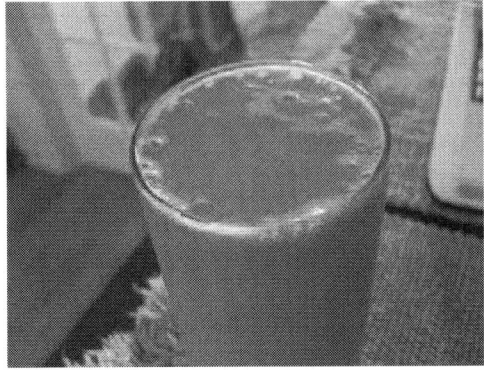

Preparation Time: 20 minutes
Cooking Time: 5 minutes
Servings: 2
Ingredients:
- 2 cups of instant coffee
- 1 cup almond milk (or coconut milk)
- ¼ cup heavy cream
- 2 Tbsp. cocoa powder (unsweetened)
- 10 drops liquid stevia

Directions:
1. Make a coffee; set aside.
2. Place all remaining ingredients in your fast-speed blender; blend for 45 - 60 seconds or until done.
3. Pour your instant coffee into a blender and continue to blend for a further 30 - 45 seconds.
4. Serve immediately.

Nutrition:
- Calories: 142
- Carbohydrates: 6 g
- Proteins: 5 g
- Fat: 14 g
- Fiber: 3 g

308. Keto Blood Sugar Adjuster Smoothie

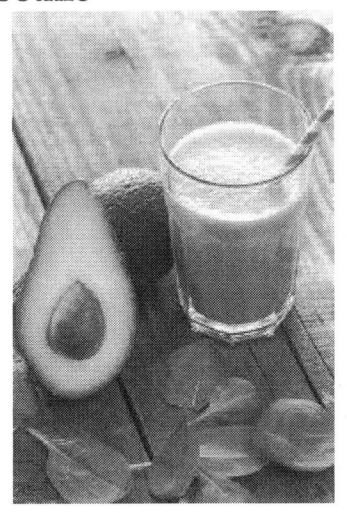

Preparation Time: 10 minutes
Cooking Time: 5 minutes
Servings: 2 servings
Ingredients:
- 2 cups of green cabbage
- 1 Tbsp. Apple cider vinegar
- Juice of 1 small lemon
- 1 cup of water
- 1 cup of crushed ice cubes for serving.

Directions:
1. Place all ingredients in your high-speed blender or a food processor and blend until smooth and soft.
2. Serve in chilled glasses with crushed ice.
3. Enjoy!

Nutrition:
- Calories: 74
- Carbohydrates: 7 g
- Proteins: 2 g
- Fat: 6 g Fiber: 4 g

309. Lime Smoothie

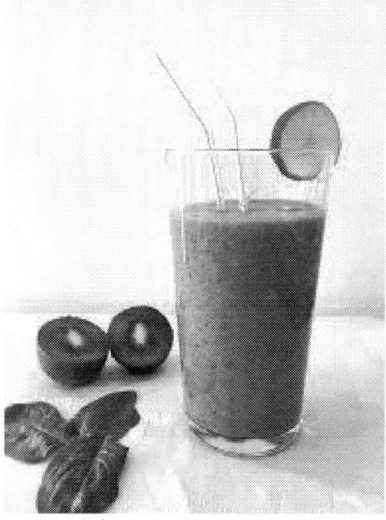

Preparation Time: 5 minutes
Cooking Time: 5 minutes
Servings: 2 servings
Ingredients:
- 1 cup water
- 1 lime juice (2 limes)
- 1 green apple cut into chunks; core discarded
- ½ cup fresh chopped fresh mint
- Ice crushed
- ¼ tsp ground cinnamon
- 1 Tbsp. natural sweetener of your choice (optional)

Directions:
1. Place all ingredients in your high-speed blender.
2. Blend for 45 - 60 seconds or until your smoothie is smooth and creamy.
3. Serve in a chilled glass.
4. Adjust sweetener to taste.

Nutrition:
- Calories: 112
- Carbohydrates: 8 g
- Proteins: 4 g
- Fat: 10 g
- Fiber: 5.5 g

310. Protein Coconut Smoothie

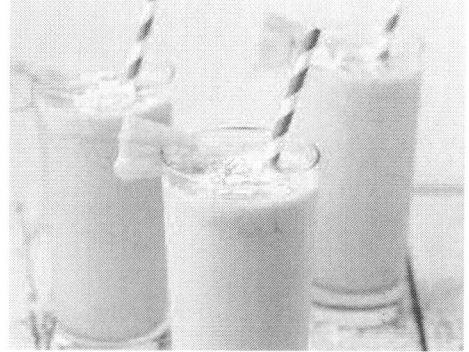

Preparation Time: 15 minutes
Cooking Time: 5 minutes
Servings: 2
Ingredients:
- 1 ½ cup of coconut milk
- 1 scoop vanilla protein powder
- 2 Tbsp. chia seeds
- 1 cup of ice cubes crushed
- 2 - 3 Tbsp. Stevia granulated natural sweetener (optional)

Directions:
1. Place all ingredients from the list above in a blender.

2. Blend until you get a smoothie-like consistently.
3. Serve into a chilled glass, and it is ready to drink.

Nutrition:
- Calories: 377 Carbohydrates: 7 g
- Proteins: 10 g Fat: 38 g
- Fiber: 2 g

311. Total Almond Smoothie
Preparation Time: 15 minutes
Cooking Time: 5 minutes
Servings: 2
Ingredients:
- 1 ½ cups of almond milk
- 2 tbsp. of almond butter
- 2 tbsp. ground almonds
- 1 cup of fresh kale leave s (or to taste)
- ½ tsp of cocoa powder
- 1 tbsp. chia seeds
- ½ cup of water

Directions:
1. Rinse and carefully clean kale leaves from any dirt.
2. Add almond milk, almond butter, and ground almonds in your blender; blend for 45 - 60 seconds.
3. Add kale leaves, cocoa powder, and chia seeds; blend for further 45 seconds.
4. If your smoothie is too thick, pour more almond milk or water.
5. Serve.

Nutrition:
- Calories: 228
- Carbohydrates: 7 g
- Proteins: 8 g
- Fat: 11 g
- Fiber: 6 g

312. Ultimate Green Mix Smoothie

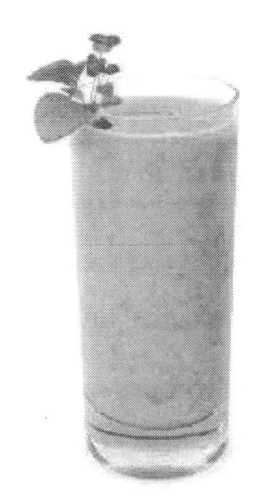

Preparation Time: 15 minutes
Cooking Time: 5 minutes
Servings: 2
Ingredients:
- Handful of collard greens
- Handful of lettuce, any kind
- 1 ½ cup of almond milk
- ½ cup of water
- ¼ cup of stevia granulated sweetener
- 1 tsp pure vanilla extract
- 1 cup crushed ice cubes (optional)

Directions:
1. Rinse and carefully clean your greens from any dirt.
2. Place all ingredients from the list above in your blender or food processor.
3. Blend until done or 45 - 30 seconds.
4. Serve with or without crushed ice.

Nutrition:
- Calories: 73 Carbohydrates: 4 g
- Proteins: 5 g Fat: 7 g
- Fiber: 1 g

313. Hot Cocoa

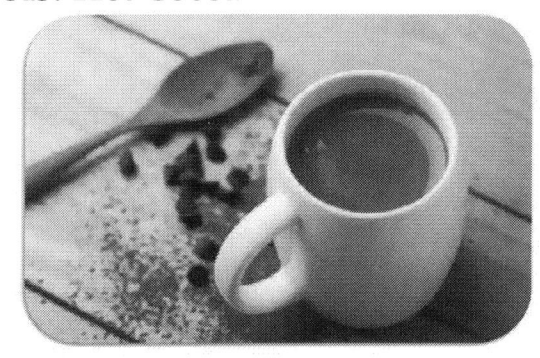

Preparation Time: 10 minutes
Cooking Time: 5 minutes
Servings: 1 serving
Ingredients:
- 1 tablespoon cocoa powder, unsweetened
- 2 teaspoons Splenda granulated sugar
- 3 tablespoons whipped dessert topping
- 1 cup water, at room temperature
- 2 tablespoons water, cold

Directions:
1. Take a saucepan, place it over medium heat, and let it heat until hot.
2. Take a cup, place cocoa powder and sugar in it, pour in cold water, and mix well.
3. Then slowly stir in hot water until the cocoa mixture dissolves and top with whipped topping.
4. Serve straight away.

Nutrition:
- Calories: 72
- Cholesterol: 0 ml
- Fat: 3 g
- Net Carbs: 1.2 g
- Protein: 1 g
- Sodium: 10 mg
- Carbohydrates: 13 g
- Potassium: 100 mg
- Fiber: 1.8 g
- Phosphorus: 49 mg

314. Cinnamon and Hazelnut Coffee

Preparation Time: 0 minutes
Cooking Time: 5 minutes
Servings: 4
Ingredients:
- 4 sticks of cinnamon
- 8 teaspoons hazelnut syrup, sugar-free
- 4 tablespoons milk, low-fat
- 4 cups brewed coffee

Directions:
1. Distribute brewed coffee into small cups, and then stir in 2 teaspoons of hazelnut syrup into each cup and 1 tablespoon milk until combined.
2. Garnish coffee with a stick of cinnamon and serve.

Nutrition:
- Calories: 13
- Cholesterol: 1 ml
- Fat: 0 g
- Net Carbs: 1 g
- Protein: 1 g
- Sodium: 13 mg
- Carbohydrates: 1 g
- Potassium: 139 mg
- Fiber: 0 g
- Phosphorus: 22 mg

315. Almond Milk

Preparation Time: 5 minutes
Cooking Time: 0 minutes
Servings: 3
Ingredient:
- 1 cup almonds, soaked in warm water for 10 minutes
- 1 teaspoon vanilla extract, unsweetened
- 3 cups of filtered water

Directions:
1. Drain the soaked almonds, place them into the blender, pour in water, and blend for 2 minutes until almonds are chopped.
2. Strain the milk by passing it through a cheesecloth into a bowl, discard almond meal, and then stir vanilla into the milk.
3. Cover the milk, refrigerate until chilled, and when ready to serve, stir it well, pour the milk evenly into the glasses and then serve.

Nutrition:
- Calories: 40 Cholesterol: 0 ml
- Fat: 3 g Net Carbs: 2 g
- Protein: 1 g
- Sodium: 6 mg
- Carbohydrates: 2 g
- Potassium: 180 mg
- Fiber: 0 g
- Phosphorus: 40 mg

316. Cucumber and Lemon-Flavored Water

Preparation Time: 3 hours and 5 minutes
Cooking Time: 0 minutes
Servings: 10
Ingredients:
- 1 lemon, deseeded, sliced
- ¼ cup fresh mint leaves, chopped
- 1 medium cucumber, sliced
- ¼ cup fresh basil leaves, chopped
- 10 cups water

Directions:
1. Take a pitcher, place all the ingredients (in order) in it, and then stir until mixed.
2. Place the pitcher in the refrigerator, chill the water for a minimum of 3 hours (or overnight), and then serve.

Nutrition:
- Calories: 4
- Cholesterol: 0 ml
- Fat: 0 g
- Net Carbs: 0.6 g
- Protein: 0 g
- Sodium: 8 mg
- Carbohydrate: 1 g
- Potassium: 38 mg
- Fiber: 0.4 g
- Phosphorus: 4 mg

CHAPTER 14:

Snacks

317. Sesame-Garlic Edamame
Preparation Time: 10 minutes
Cooking Time: 10 minutes
Servings: 4
Ingredients:
- 1 (14-ounce) package frozen edamame in their shells
- 1 tablespoon canola or sunflower oil - 1 tablespoon toasted sesame oil - 3 garlic cloves, minced
- ½ teaspoon kosher salt
- ¼ teaspoon red pepper flakes (or more)

Directions:
1. Bring a large pot of water to a boil over high heat. Add the edamame, and cook just long enough to warm them up 2 to 3 minutes.
2. Meanwhile, heat the canola oil, sesame oil, garlic, salt, and red pepper flakes in a large skillet over medium heat for 1 to 2 minutes, then remove the pan from the heat.
3. Drain the edamame and add them to the skillet, tossing to combine.

Nutrition:
- Calories: 173 Total Fat: 12 g
- Saturated Fat:1 g Cholesterol:0 mg
- Sodium: 246 mg Carbohydrates: 8 g
- Fiber: 5 g Added Sugars: 0 g
- Protein: 11 g Potassium: 487 mg
- Vitamin K: 34 mcg

318. Rosemary and White Bean Dip
Preparation Time: 10 minutes
Cooking Time: 10 minutes
Servings: 10 (¼ cup per serving)
Ingredients:
- 1 (15-ounce) can cannellini beans, rinsed and drained
- 2 tablespoons extra-virgin olive oil
- 1 garlic clove, peeled
- 1 teaspoon finely chopped fresh rosemary
- Pinch cayenne pepper
- Freshly ground black pepper
- 1 (7.5-ounce) jar marinated artichoke hearts, drained

Directions:
1. Blend the beans, oil, garlic, rosemary, cayenne pepper, and black pepper in a food processor until smooth.
2. Add the artichoke hearts, and pulse until roughly chopped but not puréed.

Nutrition:
- Calories: 75 Total Fat: 5 g
- Saturated Fat: 1 g Cholesterol: 0 mg
- Sodium: 139 mg
- Carbohydrates: 6 g Fiber: 3 g
- Added Sugars: 0 g Protein: 2 g
- Potassium: 75 mg
- Vitamin K: 1 mcg

319. Garlicky Kale Chips

Preparation Time: 5 minutes
Cooking Time: 25 minutes
Servings: 4
Ingredients:
- 1 bunch curly kale
- 2 teaspoons extra-virgin olive oil
- ¼ teaspoon kosher salt
- ¼ teaspoon garlic powder (optional)

Directions:
1. Preheat the oven to 325°F. Line a rimmed baking sheet with parchment paper.
2. Remove the tough stems from the kale, and tear the leaves into squares about big potato chips (they'll shrink when cooked).
3. Transfer the kale to a large bowl, and drizzle with the oil. Massage with your fingers for 1 to 2 minutes to coat well. Spread out on the baking sheet.
4. Cook for 8 minutes, then toss and cook for another 7 minutes and check them. Take them out as soon as they feel crispy, likely within the next 5 minutes.
5. Sprinkle with salt and garlic powder (if using). Enjoy immediately.

Nutrition:
- Calories: 28 Total Fat: 2 g
- Saturated Fat: 0 g
- Cholesterol: 0 mg
- Sodium: 126 mg
- Carbohydrates: 2 g
- Fiber: 1 g
- Added Sugars: 0 g
- Protein: 1 g
- Potassium: 81 mg
- Vitamin K: 114 mcg

320. Baked Tortilla Chips

Preparation Time: 5 minutes
Cooking Time: 20 minutes
Servings: 4
Ingredients:
- 1 tablespoon canola or sunflower oil
- 4 medium whole-wheat tortillas
- ⅛ teaspoon coarse salt

Directions:
1. Preheat the oven to 350°F.
2. Brush the oil onto both sides of each tortilla. Stack them on a large cutting board, and cut the entire stack at once, cutting the stack into 8 wedges of each tortilla. Transfer the tortilla pieces to a rimmed baking sheet. Sprinkle a little salt over each chip.
3. Bake for 10 minutes, and then flip the chips. Bake for another 3 to 5 minutes, until they're just starting to brown.

Nutrition:
- Calories: 194
- Total Fat: 11 g
- Saturated Fat: 2 g
- Cholesterol: 0 mg
- Sodium: 347 mg
- Carbohydrates: 20 g
- Fiber: 4 g
- Added Sugars: 0 g
- Protein: 4 g
- Potassium: 111 mg
- Vitamin K: 7 mcg

321. Spicy Guacamole

Preparation Time: 15 minutes
Cooking Time: 15 minutes
Servings: 4 (about 3 tablespoons per serving)
Ingredients:
- 1½ tablespoons freshly squeezed lime juice
- 1 tablespoon minced jalapeño pepper, or to taste
- 1 tablespoon minced red onion
- 1 tablespoon chopped fresh cilantro
- 1 garlic clove, minced
- ⅛ to ¼ teaspoon kosher salt
- Freshly ground black pepper

Directions:
1. Combine the lime juice, jalapeño, onion, cilantro, garlic, salt, and pepper in a large bowl, and mix well.

Nutrition:
- Calories: 61 Total Fat: 5 g
- Saturated Fat: 1 g
- Cholesterol: 0 mg
- Sodium: 123 mg
- Carbohydrates: 4 g Fiber: 2 g
- Added Sugars: 0 g Protein: 1 g
- Potassium: 195 mg
- Vitamin K: 8 mcg

322. Chickpea Fatteh

Preparation Time: 25 minutes
Cooking Time: 25 minutes
Servings: 8
Ingredients:
- 2 (4-inch) whole-wheat pitas
- 4 tablespoons extra-virgin olive oil, divided
- 1 (15-ounce) can no-salt-added chickpeas, rinsed and drained
- ⅓ cup pine nuts
- 1 cup plain 1% yogurt
- 2 garlic cloves, minced
- ¼ teaspoon salt
- ½ cup pomegranate seeds (optional)

Directions:
1. Preheat the oven to 375°F.
2. Cut the pitas into 1-inch squares (no need to separate the two halves), and toss with 2 tablespoons of oil in a large bowl. Spread onto a rimmed baking sheet and bake, occasionally shaking the sheet until golden brown, about 10 minutes.
3. Meanwhile, gently warm the chickpeas and 1 tablespoon of oil in a small saucepan over medium-low heat, 4 to 5 minutes.
4. Toast the pine nuts in a skillet with the remaining 1 tablespoon of oil over medium heat until golden brown, 4 to 5 minutes.
5. Mix the yogurt with the garlic and salt in a small bowl.
6. Transfer the toasted pitas to a wide serving bowl. Top with the chickpeas. Drizzle with the yogurt mixture, then top with the pine nuts and pomegranate seeds (if using).

Nutrition:
- Calories: 198 Total Fat: 12 g
- Saturated Fat: 2 g
- Cholesterol: 2 mg
- Sodium: 144 mg
- Carbohydrates: 18 g Fiber: 3 g
- Added Sugars: 0 g Protein: 6 g
- Potassium: 236 mg
- Vitamin K: 9 mcg

323. Marinated Berries
Preparation Time: 5 minutes
Cooking Time: 30 minutes
Servings: 4
Ingredients:
- 2 cups fresh strawberries, hulled and quartered
- 1 cup fresh blueberries (optional)
- 2 tablespoons sugar
- 1 tablespoon balsamic vinegar
- 2 tablespoons chopped fresh mint (optional)
- ⅛ teaspoon freshly ground black pepper

Directions:
1. Gently toss the strawberries, blueberries (if using), sugar, vinegar, mint (if using), and pepper in a large nonreactive bowl.
2. Let the flavors blend for at least 25 minutes, or as long as 2 hours.

Nutrition:
- Calories: 73 Total Fat: 8 g
- Saturated Fat: 8 g
- Cholesterol: 0 mg
- Sodium: 4 mg
- Carbohydrates: 18 g
- Fiber: 2 g
- Added Sugars: 6 g
- Protein: 1 g
- Potassium: 162 mg
- Vitamin K: 9 mcg

324. Pumpkin-Turmeric Latte
Preparation Time: 10 minutes
Cooking Time: 10 minutes
Servings: 1
Ingredients:
- ½ cup brewed espresso or 1 cup brewed strong coffee
- ¼ cup pumpkin purée
- 1 teaspoon vanilla extract
- 1 teaspoon sugar
- ½ teaspoon ground turmeric
- ½ teaspoon ground cinnamon, plus more if needed
- 1 cup 1% milk

Directions:
1. Combine the espresso, pumpkin, vanilla, sugar, turmeric, and cinnamon in a medium saucepan over medium heat, whisking occasionally.
2. Warm the milk over low heat in a small pan. When it is warm (not hot), whisk it vigorously (or mix with a blender or handheld frother) to make it foamy.
3. Pour the hot coffee mixture into a mug, then top with the frothy milk. Sprinkle with more cinnamon, if desired.

Nutrition:
- Calories: 169 Total Fat: 3 g
- Saturated Fat: 2 g
- Cholesterol: 12 mg
- Sodium: 128 mg
- Carbohydrates: 26 g
- Fiber: 3 g
- Added Sugars: 5 g
- Protein: 9 g
- Potassium: 665 mg
- Vitamin K: 11 mcg

325. Dark Hot Chocolate
Preparation Time: 5 minutes
Cooking Time: 5 minutes
Servings: 2
Ingredients:
- 1¾ cups vanilla soy milk

- 1-ounce dark chocolate (70% cacao or more), broken into small pieces

Directions:
1. Heat the soy milk in a small saucepan over medium-high heat and add the chocolate. When the milk starts bubbling, turn the heat to low.
2. Whisk until the chocolate is melted and fully incorporated. Tip the pot to make sure there is no remaining chocolate on the bottom.

Nutrition:
- Calories: 149
- Total Fat: 8 g
- Saturated Fat: 3 g
- Cholesterol: 0 mg
- Sodium: 105 mg
- Carbohydrates: 14 g
- Fiber: 2 g
- Added Sugars: 5 g
- Protein: 6 g
- Potassium: 351 mg
- Vitamin K: 4 mcg

326. Dark Chocolate and Cherry Trail Mix

Preparation Time: 5 minutes
Cooking Time: 5 minutes
Servings: Makes 3 cups (¼ cup per serving)
Ingredients:
- 1 cup unsalted almonds
- ⅔ cup dried cherries
- ½ cup walnuts
- ½ cup sweet cinnamon-roasted chickpeas
- ¼ cup dark chocolate chips

Directions:
1. Combine the almonds, cherries, walnuts, chickpeas, and chocolate chips in an airtight container.
2. Store at room temperature for up to 1 week or in the freezer for up to 3 months.

Nutrition:
- Calories: 174
- Total Fat: 12 g
- Saturated Fat: 2 g
- Cholesterol: 0 mg
- Sodium: 18 mg
- Carbohydrates: 16 g
- Fiber: 4 g
- Added Sugars: 7 g
- Protein: 5 g
- Potassium: 134 mg
- Vitamin K: 0 mcg

327. Happy Heart Energy Bites

Preparation Time: 20 minutes
Cooking Time: 30 min
Servings: Makes 30 (2 balls per serving)
Ingredients:
- 1 cup rolled oats
- ¾ cup chopped walnuts
- ½ cup natural peanut butter
- ½ cup ground flaxseed
- ¼ cup honey
- ¼ cup dried cranberries

Directions:
1. Combine the oats, walnuts, peanut butter, flaxseed, honey, and cranberries in a large bowl.
2. Refrigerate for 10 to 20 minutes, if you can, to make them easier to roll.

3. Roll into ¾-inch balls. Store in the fridge or freezer, if they don't disappear first.

Nutrition:
- Calories: 174
- Total Fat: 10 g
- Saturated Fat: 1 g
- Cholesterol: 0 mg
- Sodium: 43 mg
- Carbohydrates: 17 g
- Fiber: 3 g
- Added Sugars: 7 g
- Protein: 5 g
- Potassium: 169 mg
- Vitamin K: 1 mcg

328. Chocolate-Cashew Spread

Preparation Time: 10 minutes
Cooking Time: 10 minutes
Servings: Makes ½ cup (2 tablespoons per serving)

Ingredients:
- ¼ cup unsalted cashew butter
- 3 tablespoons water
- 1½ tablespoons unsweetened cocoa powder
- 2 teaspoons honey
- 1 teaspoon extra-virgin olive oil
- ½ teaspoon vanilla extract
- Pinch of ground cinnamon
- Pinch of salt

Directions:
1. Stir together the cashew butter, water, cocoa powder, honey, olive oil, vanilla, cinnamon, and salt in a large bowl until smooth, 2 to 3 minutes.

Nutrition:
- Calories: 108
- Total Fat: 9 g
- Saturated Fat: 2 g
- Cholesterol: 0 mg
- Sodium: 93 mg
- Carbohydrates: 8 g
- Fiber: 1 g
- Added Sugars: 3 g
- Protein: 2 g
- Potassium: 92 mg
- Vitamin K: 5 mcg

329. Mango Chiller

Preparation Time: 5 minutes
Cooking Time: 5 minutes
Servings: 4 (½ cup per serving)

Ingredients:
- 2 cups frozen mango chunks
- ½ cup plain 2% Greek yogurt
- ¼ cup 1% milk
- 2 teaspoons honey (optional)

Directions:
1. Mix the mango and yogurt in a food processor or blender. Add the milk, a bit at a time, to get it to soft ice cream consistency.
2. Taste, and add honey if you like. Enjoy immediately.

Nutrition:
- Calories: 85
- Total Fat: 1 g
- Saturated Fat: 1 g
- Cholesterol: 4 mg
- Sodium: 17 mg
- Carbohydrates: 16 g
- Fiber: 1 g
- Added Sugars: 3 g
- Protein: 4 g
- Potassium: 197 mg
- Vitamin K: 3 mcg

330. Blueberry-Ricotta Swirl

Preparation Time: 5 minutes
Cooking Time: 5 minutes
Servings: 2
Ingredients:
- ½ cup fresh or frozen blueberries
- ½ cup part-skim ricotta cheese
- 1 teaspoon sugar
- ½ teaspoon lemon zest (optional)

Directions:
1. If using frozen blueberries, warm them in a saucepan over medium heat until they are thawed but not hot.
2. Meanwhile, mix the sugar with the ricotta in a medium bowl.
3. Mix the blueberries into the ricotta, leaving a few out. Taste, and add more sugar if desired. Top with the remaining blueberries and lemon zest (if using).

Nutrition:
- Calories: 113 Total Fat: 5 g
- Saturated Fat: 3 g
- Cholesterol: 19 mg
- Sodium: 62 mg
- Carbohydrates: 10 g
- Fiber: 1 g
- Added Sugars: 2 g
- Protein: 7 g
- Potassium: 98 mg
- Vitamin K: 7 mcg

331. Roasted Broccoli and Cauliflower

Preparation Time: 7 minutes
Cooking Time: 23 minutes
Servings: 6
Ingredients:
- 2 cups broccoli florets
- 2 cups cauliflower florets
- 2 tablespoons olive oil
- 1 tablespoon freshly squeezed lemon juice
- 2 teaspoons Dijon mustard
- ¼ teaspoon garlic powder
- Pinch salt
- 1/8 teaspoon freshly ground black pepper

Directions:
1. Preheat the oven to 425°F.
2. On a baking sheet with a lip, combine the broccoli and cauliflower florets in one even layer.
3. In a small bowl, combine the olive oil, lemon juice, mustard, garlic powder, salt, and pepper until well blended and drizzle the mixture over the vegetables. Toss to coat and spread the vegetables out in a single layer again.
4. Roast for 22 minutes. Serve immediately.

Nutrition:
- Calories: 63
- Sodium: 74 mg
- Phosphorus: 39 mg
- Potassium: 216 mg
- Protein: 2 g

332. Herbed Garlic Cauliflower Mash

Preparation Time: 10 minutes
Cooking Time: 20 minutes
Servings: 6
Ingredients:
- 4 cups cauliflower florets
- 4 garlic cloves, peeled
- 4 ounces cream cheese, softened
- ¼ cup unsweetened almond milk

- 2 tablespoons unsalted butter
- Pinch salt
- 2 tablespoons minced fresh chives
- 2 tablespoons chopped flat-leaf parsley
- 1 tablespoon fresh thyme leaves

Directions:
1. Boil water at high heat. Add the cauliflower and garlic and cook, occasionally stirring until the cauliflower is tender, about 8 to 10 minutes.
2. Drain the cauliflower and garlic into a colander in the sink and shake the colander well to remove excess water.
3. Using a paper towel, blot the vegetables to remove any remaining water. Return the florets to the pot and place over low heat for 1 minute to remove as much water as possible.
4. Mash the florets and garlic with a potato masher until smooth.
5. Beat in the cream cheese, almond milk, butter, salt, chives, parsley, and thyme with a spoon. Serve.

Nutrition:
- Calories: 124
- Sodium: 115 mg
- Phosphorus: 59 mg
- Potassium: 266 mg
- Protein: 3 g

333. Sautéed Spicy Cabbage

Preparation Time: 15 minutes
Cooking Time: 5 minutes
Servings: 6
Ingredients:
- 3 tablespoons olive oil
- 3 cups chopped green cabbage
- 3 cups chopped red cabbage
- 2 garlic cloves, minced
- 1/8 teaspoon cayenne pepper
- Pinch salt

Directions:
1. Cook olive oil in a large skillet over medium heat.
2. Stir in red and green cabbage and garlic; sauté until the leaves wilt and are tender for about 4 to 5 minutes.
3. Sprinkle the vegetables with the cayenne pepper and salt, toss, and serve.

Nutrition:
- Calories: 86
- Sodium: 46 mg
- Phosphorus: 27 mg
- Potassium: 189 mg
- Protein: 1 g

334. Fragrant Thai-Style Eggplant

Preparation Time: 10 minutes
Cooking Time: 20 minutes
Servings: 6
Ingredients:
- 1 eggplant, cut into ½-inch slices
- ¼ teaspoon salt
- 1 tablespoon extra-virgin olive oil
- 1 tablespoon peeled and grated fresh ginger root
- 1 garlic clove, minced
- 2 tablespoons freshly squeezed lime juice
- 1 tablespoon water
- 2 tablespoons chopped fresh basil

Directions:
1. Preheat the oven to 400°F.
2. On a baking sheet with a lip, arrange the eggplant slices and sprinkle evenly with the salt. Drizzle with the olive oil.

3. Bake the eggplant for 10 minutes, then remove the baking sheet from the oven and turn the slices over. Return the baking sheet to the oven and bake for 10 to 15 minutes longer or until the eggplant is tender.
4. Meanwhile, stir together the ginger, garlic, lime juice, water, and basil in a small bowl until well mixed.
5. Situate the eggplant on a serving plate and drizzle with the ginger mixture. Serve warm or cool.

Nutrition:
- Calories: 52
- Sodium: 101 mg
- Phosphorus: 30 mg
- Potassium: 280 mg
- Protein: 1 g

335. Roasted Asparagus with Pine Nuts

Preparation Time: 10 minutes
Cooking Time: 13 minutes
Servings: 4
Ingredients:
- 1-pound fresh asparagus, woody ends removed
- 1 tablespoon olive oil
- 1 tablespoon balsamic vinegar
- 3 garlic cloves, minced
- ½ teaspoon dried thyme leaves
- ¼ cup pine nuts

Directions:
1. Preheat the oven to 400°F.
2. Rinse the asparagus and arrange in a single layer on a baking sheet.
3. Blend olive oil, balsamic vinegar, garlic, and thyme until well mixed.
4. Drizzle the dressing over the asparagus and toss to coat.
5. Roast the asparagus for 10 minutes and remove the baking sheet from the oven.
6. Sprinkle the pine nuts over the asparagus and return the baking sheet to the oven. Roast for another 5 to 7 minutes or until the pine nuts are toasted and the asparagus is tender and light golden brown. Serve.

Nutrition:
- Calories: 116
- Sodium: 4 mg
- Phosphorus: 112 mg
- Potassium: 294 mg
- Protein: 4 g

336. Roasted Radishes

Preparation Time: 10 minutes
Cooking Time: 20 minutes
Servings: 6
Ingredients:
- 3 bunches whole small radishes
- 3 tablespoons olive oil, divided
- 1 tablespoon freshly squeezed lemon juice
- 1 tablespoon Dijon mustard
- ½ teaspoon dried marjoram leaves
- 1/8 teaspoon white pepper
- Pinch salt
- 2 tablespoons chopped flat-leaf parsley

Directions:
1. Preheat the oven to 425°F. Prep a baking sheet with a lip with parchment paper and set aside.
2. Scrub the radishes, remove the stem and root, and cut each in half or thirds, depending on the size. The radishes should be similarly sized, so they cook evenly.

3. Toss the radishes and 1 tablespoon olive oil on the baking sheet to coat and arrange the radishes in a single layer.
4. Roast the radishes for 18 to 20 minutes or until they are lightly golden and tender but still crisp on the outside.
5. While the radishes are roasting, whisk together the remaining 2 tablespoons of olive oil with the lemon juice, mustard, marjoram, pepper, and salt in a small bowl.
6. Once done, take them from the baking sheet and place them in a serving bowl. Drizzle the vegetables with the dressing and toss. Sprinkle with the parsley. Serve warm or cool.

Nutrition:
- Calories: 79
- Sodium: 123 mg
- Phosphorus: 23 mg
- Potassium: 232 mg
- Protein: 1 g

337. Grilled Peppers in Chipotle Vinaigrette

Preparation Time: 15 minutes
Cooking Time: 6 minutes
Servings: 4
Ingredients:
- 1 red bell pepper
- 1 yellow bell pepper
- 1 orange bell pepper
- 2 tablespoons extra-virgin olive oil
- Juice of 1 lemon
- 1 tsp. minced chipotle peppers in adobo sauce

Directions:
1. Prepare and preheat the grill to medium coals and set a grill 6 inches from the coals. If grilling indoors, heat the grill pan over medium-high heat. For charcoal grills, medium coals mean you can hold your palm 6 inches above the grill rack for 3 to 4 seconds before you have to take it away. For gas and propane grills, medium coals are 350°F to 375°F.
2. Wash the bell peppers, remove the seeds, and cut them into 1-inch strips.
3. Blend olive oil, lemon juice, and chipotle peppers in adobo sauce.
4. Place the peppers on the grill and brush with some of the sauce. Grill the peppers for 2 to 3 minutes per side, brushing with the sauce occasionally, until the vegetables are tender and have defined grill marks. Serve.

Nutrition:
- Calories: 66
- Sodium: 90 mg
- Phosphorus: 22 mg
- Potassium: 201 mg
- Protein: 1 g

338. Double Corn Muffins

Preparation Time: 10 minutes
Cooking Time: 20 minutes
Servings: 6
Ingredients:
- ¾ cup all-purpose flour
- ¼ cup yellow cornmeal
- 2 tablespoons brown sugar
- 1 teaspoon cream of tartar
- ½ teaspoon baking soda
- Pinch salt

- 1 large egg
- ½ cup unsweetened almond milk
- ½ cup whole kernel corn
- 3 tablespoons unsalted butter, melted

Directions:
1. Preheat the oven to 350°F. Prep a 6-cup muffin pan with paper liners and set aside.
2. Scourge flour, cornmeal, brown sugar, cream of tartar, baking soda, and salt until well blended.
3. In a small bowl, stir together the egg, milk, corn, and melted butter.
4. Add the liquid ingredients to the dry ingredients and stir just until combined.
5. Split the batter among the prepared muffin cups, filling each about ¾ full.
6. Bake for 18 to 20 minutes or until the muffins are set and light golden brown.
7. Remove the muffins from the muffin tin and set on a wire rack to cool. Serve warm.

Nutrition:
- Calories: 165
- Sodium: 160 mg
- Phosphorus: 55 mg
- Potassium: 168 mg
- Protein: 4 g

CHAPTER 15:

Desserts

339. Spiced Peaches

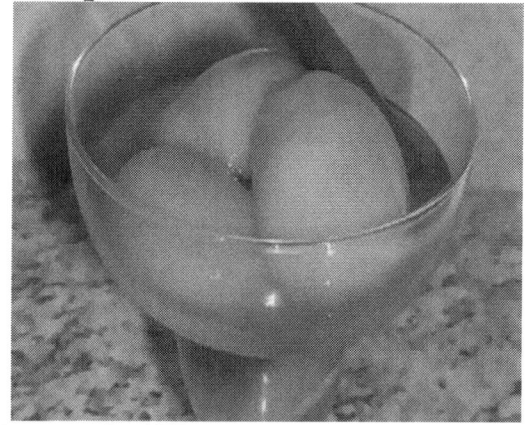

Preparation Time: 5 minutes
Cooking Time: 10 minutes
Servings: 2
Ingredients:
- 1 cup Peaches
- ½ tsp Cornstarch
- 1 tsp Ground cloves
- 1 tsp Ground cinnamon
- 1 tsp Ground nutmeg
- Zest of ½ lemon
- ½ cup Water

Directions:
1. Combine cinnamon, cornstarch, nutmeg, ground cloves, and lemon zest in a pan on the stove.
2. Heat on medium heat and add peaches.
3. Bring to a boil, reduce the heat and simmer for 10 minutes.
4. Serve.

Nutrition:
- Calories: 70 Fat: 0 g
- Carbs: 14 g Phosphorus: 23 mg
- Potassium: 176 mg
- Sodium: 3 mg
- Protein: 1 g

340. Pumpkin Cheesecake Bar

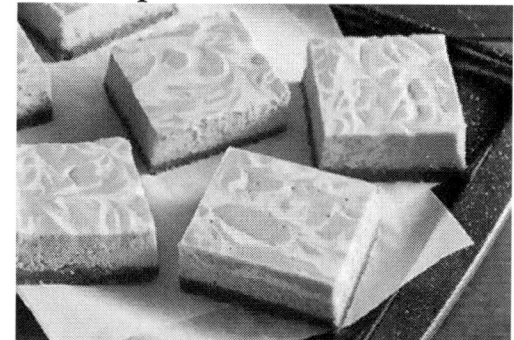

Preparation Time: 10 minutes
Cooking Time: 50 minutes
Servings: 4
Ingredients:
- 2 ½ tbsps Unsalted butter
- 4 oz. Cream cheese
- ½ cup All-purpose white flour
- 3 tbsps Golden brown sugar
- ¼ cup Granulated sugar
- ½ cup Pureed pumpkin
- 2 Egg whites
- 1 tsp Ground cinnamon
- 1 tsp Ground nutmeg
- 1 tsp Vanilla extract

Directions:
1. Preheat the oven to 350F.
2. Mix flour and brown sugar in a bowl.
3. Mix in the butter to form 'breadcrumbs.'
4. Place ¾ of this mixture in a dish.
5. Bake in the oven for 15 minutes. Remove and cool.
6. Lightly whisk the egg and fold in the cream cheese, sugar, pumpkin, cinnamon, nutmeg, and vanilla until smooth.
7. Pour this mixture over the oven-baked base and sprinkle with the rest of the breadcrumbs from earlier.
8. Bake in the oven for 30 to 35 minutes more.
9. Cool, slice, and serve.

Nutrition:
- Calories: 248 Fat: 13 g
- Carbs: 33 g Phosphorus: 67 mg
- Potassium: 96 mg
- Sodium: 146 mg
- Protein: 4 g

341. Blueberry Mini Muffins

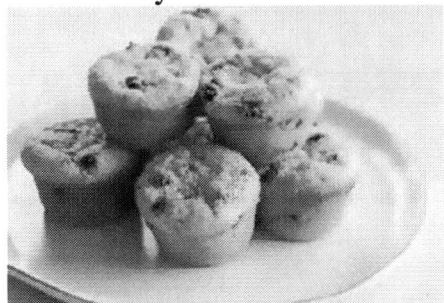

Preparation Time: 10 minutes
Cooking Time: 35 minutes
Servings: 4
Ingredients:
- 3 Egg whites
- ¼ cup All-purpose white flour
- 1 tbsp. Coconut flour
- 1 tsp. Baking soda
- 1 tbsp. Nutmeg, grated
- 1 tsp. Vanilla extract
- 1 tsp. Stevia
- ¼ cup Fresh blueberries

Directions:
1. Preheat the oven to 325F.
2. Mix all the ingredients in a bowl.
3. Divide the batter into 4 and spoon into a lightly oiled muffin tin.
4. Bake in the oven for 15 to 20 minutes or until cooked through.
5. Cool and serve.

Nutrition:
- Calories: 62 Fat: 0 g
- Carbs: 9 g Phosphorus: 103 mg
- Potassium: 65 mg
- Sodium: 62 mg Protein: 4 g

342. Baked Peaches with Cream Cheese

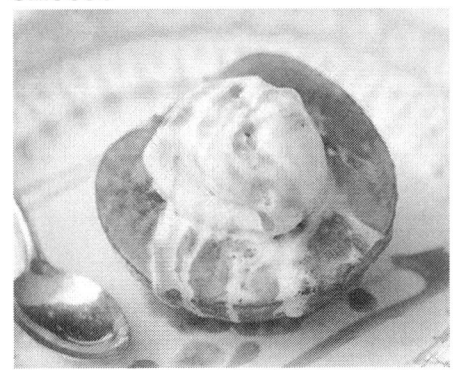

Preparation Time: 10 minutes
Cooking Time: 15 minutes
Servings: 4
Ingredients:
- 1 cup Plain cream cheese
- ½ cup Crushed meringue cookies
- ¼ tsp Ground cinnamon

- Pinch ground nutmeg
- 8 peach halves
- 2 tbsp. Honey

Directions:
1. Preheat the oven to 350F.
2. Line a baking sheet with parchment paper. Set aside.
3. In a small bowl, stir together the meringue cookies, cream cheese, cinnamon, and nutmeg.
4. Spoon the cream cheese mixture evenly into the cavities in the peach halves.
5. Place the peaches on the baking sheet and bake for 15 minutes or until the fruit is soft and the cheese is melted.
6. Remove the peaches from the baking sheet onto plates.
7. Drizzle with honey and serve.

Nutrition:
- Calories: 260 Fat: 20
- Carbs: 19 g Phosphorus: 74 mg
- Potassium: 198 mg
- Sodium: 216 mg Protein: 4 g

343. Bread Pudding

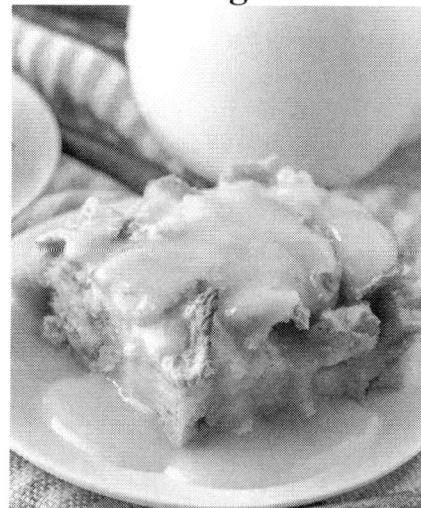

Preparation Time: 15 minutes
Cooking Time: 40 minutes
Servings: 6
Ingredients:
- Unsalted butter, for greasing the baking dish
- 1 ½ cups Plain rice milk
- 2 Eggs
- 2 Egg whites
- ¼ cup Honey
- 1 tsp. Pure vanilla extract
- 6 cups Cubed white bread

Directions:
1. Lightly grease an 8-by-8-inch baking dish with butter. Set aside.
2. In a bowl, whisk together the eggs, egg whites, rice milk, honey, and vanilla.
3. Add the bread cubes and stir until the bread is coated.
4. Transfer the mixture to the baking dish and cover with plastic wrap.
5. Store the dish in the refrigerator for at least 3 hours.
6. Preheat the oven to 325F.
7. Remove the plastic wrap from the baking dish, bake the pudding for 35 to 40 minutes, or golden brown.
8. Serve.

Nutrition:
- Calories: 167
- Fat: 3 g
- Carbs: 30 g
- Phosphorus: 95 mg
- Potassium: 93 mg
- Sodium: 189 mg
- Protein: 6 g

344. Strawberry Ice Cream

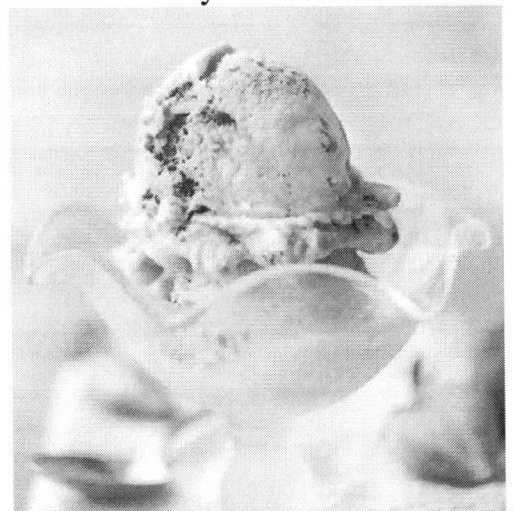

Preparation Time: 5 minutes
Cooking Time: 5 minutes
Servings: 3
Ingredients:
- ½ cup Stevia
- 1 tbsp Lemon juice
- ¾ cup Non-dairy coffee creamer
- 10 oz. Strawberries
- 1 cup Crushed ice

Directions:
1. Blend everything in a blender until smooth.
2. Freeze until frozen.
3. Serve.

Nutrition:
- Calories: 94.4
- Fat: 6 g
- Carbs: 8.3 g
- Phosphorus: 25 mg
- Potassium: 108 mg
- Sodium: 25 mg
- Protein: 1.3 g

345. Cinnamon Custard

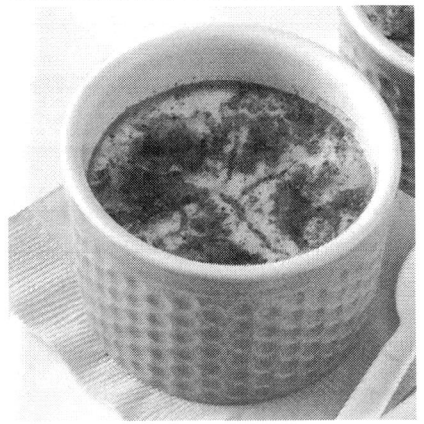

Preparation Time: 20 minutes
Cooking Time: 1 hour
Servings: 6
Ingredients:
- Unsalted butter, for greasing the ramekins
- 1 ½ cups Plain rice milk
- 4 Eggs
- ¼ cup Granulated sugar
- 1 tsp. Pure vanilla extract
- ½ tsp. Ground cinnamon
- Cinnamon sticks for garnish

Directions:
1. Preheat the oven to 325F.
2. Lightly grease 6 ramekins and place them in a baking dish. Set aside.
3. In a large bowl, whisk together the eggs, rice milk, sugar, vanilla, and cinnamon until the mixture is smooth.
4. Pour the mixture through a fine sieve into a pitcher.
5. Evenly divide the custard mixture among the ramekins.
    Fill the baking dish with hot water until the water reaches halfway up the ramekins' sides.

6. Bake for 1 hour or until the custards are set, and a knife inserted in the center comes out clean.
7. Remove the custards from the oven and take the ramekins out of the water.
8. Cool on the wire racks for 1 hour, then chill for 1 hour.
9. Garnish with cinnamon sticks and serve.

Nutrition:
- Calories: 110
- Fat: 4 g
- Carbs: 14 g
- Phosphorus: 100 mg
- Potassium: 64 mg
- Sodium: 71 mg
- Protein: 4 g

346. Raspberry Brule

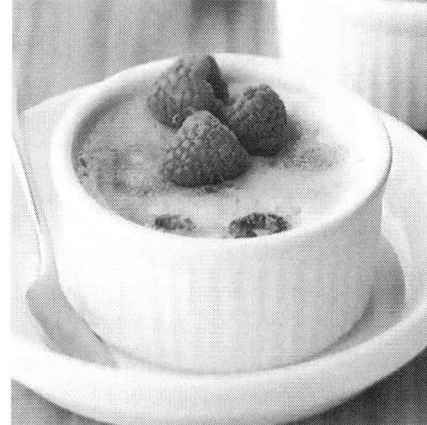

Preparation Time: 15 minutes
Cooking Time: 1 minute
Servings: 4
Ingredients:
- ½ cup Light sour cream
- ½ cup Plain cream cheese
- ¼ cup Brown sugar, divided
- ¼ tsp. Ground cinnamon
- 1 cup Fresh raspberries

Directions:
1. Preheat the oven to broil.
2. In a bowl, beat together the cream cheese, sour cream, 2 tbsp. brown sugar and cinnamon for 4 minutes or until the mixture is very smooth and fluffy.
3. Evenly divide the raspberries among 4 (4-ounce) ramekins.
4. Spoon the cream cheese mixture over the berries and smooth the tops.
5. Sprinkle ½ tbsp. brown sugar evenly over each ramekin.
6. Place the ramekins on a baking sheet and broil 4 inches from the heating element until the sugar is caramelized and golden brown.
7. Cool and serve.

Nutrition:
- Calories: 188
- Fat: 13 g
- Carbs: 16 g
- Phosphorus: 60 mg
- Potassium: 158 mg
- Sodium: 132 mg

347. Tart Apple Granita

Preparation Time: 15 minutes, plus 4 hours freezing time
Cooking Time: 0 minutes
Servings: 4
Ingredients:
- ½ cup granulated sugar
- ½ cup water
- 2 cups unsweetened apple juice
- ¼ cup freshly squeezed lemon juice

Directions:
1. In a small saucepan over medium-high heat, heat the sugar and water.

2. Bring the mixture to a boil and then reduce the heat to low and simmer for about 15 minutes or until the liquid has reduced by half.
3. Remove the pan from the heat and pour the liquid into a large shallow metal pan.
4. Let the liquid cool for about 30 minutes, and then stir in the apple juice and lemon juice.
5. Place the pan in the freezer.
6. After 1 hour, run a fork through the liquid to break up any ice crystals formed. Scrape down the sides as well.
7. Place the pan back in the freezer and repeat the stirring and scraping every 20 minutes, creating slush.
8. Serve when the mixture is completely frozen and looks like crushed ice, after about 3 hours.

Nutrition:
- Calories: 157
- Fat: 0 g
- Carbohydrates: 0 g
- Phosphorus: 10 mg
- Potassium: 141 mg
- Sodium: 5 mg
- Protein: 0 g

348. Lemon-lime Sherbet

Preparation Time: 5 minutes, plus 3 hours chilling time
Cooking Time: 15 minutes
Servings: 2
Ingredients:
- 2 cups water
- 1 cup granulated sugar
- 3 tablespoons lemon zest, divided
- ½ cup freshly squeezed lemon juice
- Zest of 1 lime
- Juice of 1 lime
- ½ cup heavy (whipping) cream

Directions:
1. Place a large saucepan over medium-high heat and add the water, sugar, and 2 tablespoons of the lemon zest.
2. Bring the mixture to a boil and then reduce the heat and simmer for 15 minutes.
3. Transfer the mixture to a large bowl and add the remaining 1 tablespoon lemon zest, the lemon juice, lime zest, and lime juice.
4. Chill the mixture in the fridge until completely cold, about 3 hours.
5. Whisk in the heavy cream and transfer the mixture to an ice cream maker.
6. Freeze according to the manufacturer's instructions.

Nutrition:
- Calories: 151
- Fat: 6 g
- Carbohydrates: 26 g
- Phosphorus: 10 mg
- Potassium: 27 mg
- Sodium: 6 mg
- Protein: 0 g

349. Pavlova with Peaches

Preparation Time: 30 minutes
Cooking Time: 1 hour, plus cooling time
Servings: 3
Ingredients:
- 4 large egg whites, at room temperature
- ½ teaspoon cream of tartar
- 1 cup superfine sugar
- ½ teaspoon pure vanilla extract
- 2 cups peaches

Directions:
1. Preheat the oven to 225°F.
2. Line a baking sheet with parchment paper; set aside.
3. In a large bowl, beat the egg whites for about 1 minute or until soft peaks form.
4. Beat in the cream of tartar.
5. Add the sugar, 1 tablespoon at a time, until the egg whites are very stiff and glossy. Do not overbeat.
6. Beat in the vanilla.
7. Evenly spoon the meringue onto the baking sheet so that you have 8 rounds.
8. Use the back of the spoon to create an indentation in the middle of each round.
9. Bake the meringues for about 1 hour or until a light brown crust forms.
10. Turn off the oven and let the meringues stand, still in the oven, overnight.
11. Remove the meringues from the sheet and place them on serving plates.
12. Spoon the peaches, dividing evenly, into the centers of the meringues, and serve.
13. Store any unused meringues in a sealed container at room temperature for up to 1 week.

Nutrition:
- Calories: 132
- Fat: 0 g
- Carbohydrates: 32 g
- Phosphorus: 7 mg
- Potassium: 95 mg
- Sodium: 30 mg
- Protein: 2 g

350. Tropical Vanilla Snow Cone

Preparation Time: 15 minutes, plus freezing time
Cooking Time: 0 minutes
Servings: 2

Ingredients:
- 1 cup pineapple
- 1 cup frozen strawberries
- 6 tablespoons water
- 2 tablespoons granulated sugar
- 1 tablespoon vanilla extract

Directions:
1. In a large saucepan, mix the peaches, pineapple, strawberries, water, and sugar over medium-high heat and bring to a boil.
2. Reduce the heat to low and simmer the mixture, occasionally stirring for about 15 minutes.
3. Remove from the heat and let the mixture cool completely, for about 1 hour.
4. Stir in the vanilla and transfer the fruit mixture to a food processor or blender.
5. Purée until smooth, and pour the purée into a 9-by-13-inch glass baking dish.
6. Cover and place the dish in the freezer overnight.
7. When the fruit mixture is completely frozen, use a fork to scrape the sorbet until you have flaked flavored ice.
8. Scoop the ice flakes into 4 serving dishes.

Nutrition:
- Calories: 92 Fat: 0 g
- Carbohydrates: 22 g
- Phosphorus: 17 mg
- Potassium: 145 mg Sodium: 4 mg
- Protein: 1 g

351. Rhubarb Crumble

Preparation Time: 15 minutes
Cooking Time: 30 minutes
Servings: 6
Ingredients:
- Unsalted butter, for greasing the baking dish
- 1 cup all-purpose flour
- ½ cup brown sugar
- ½ teaspoon ground cinnamon
- ½ cup unsalted butter, at room temperature
- 1 cup chopped rhubarb
- 2 apples, peeled, cored, and sliced thin
- 2 tablespoons granulated sugar
- 2 tablespoons water

Directions:
1. Preheat the oven to 325°F.
2. Lightly grease an 8-by-8-inch baking dish with butter; set aside.
3. In a small bowl, stir together the flour, sugar, and cinnamon until well combined.
4. Add the butter and rub the mixture between your fingers until it resembles coarse crumbs.
5. In a medium saucepan, mix the rhubarb, apple, sugar, and water over medium heat and cook for about 20 minutes or until the rhubarb is soft.
6. Spoon the fruit mixture into the baking dish and evenly top with the crumble.
7. Bake the crumble for 20 to 30 minutes or until golden brown.
8. Serve hot.

Nutrition:
- Calories: 450
- Fat: 23 g
- Carbohydrates: 60 g
- Phosphorus: 51 mg
- Potassium: 181 mg
- Sodium: 10 mg
- Protein: 4 g

352. Gingerbread Loaf

Preparation Time: 20 minutes
Cooking Time: 1 hour
Servings: 16
Ingredients:
- Unsalted butter, for greasing the baking dish
- 3 cups all-purpose flour
- ½ teaspoon Ener-G baking soda substitute
- 2 teaspoons ground cinnamon
- 1 teaspoon ground allspice
- ¾ cup granulated sugar
- 1¼ cups plain rice milk
- 1 large egg
- ¼ cup olive oil
- 2 tablespoons molasses
- 2 teaspoons grated fresh ginger
- Powdered sugar, for dusting

Directions:
1. Preheat the oven to 350°F.
2. Lightly grease a 9-by-13-inch baking dish with butter; set aside.
3. In a large bowl, sift together the flour, baking soda substitute, cinnamon, and allspice.
4. Stir the sugar into the flour mixture.
5. In a medium bowl, whisk together the milk, egg, olive oil, molasses, and ginger until well blended.
6. Make a well in the center of the flour mixture and pour in the wet ingredients.
7. Mix until just combined, taking care not to overmix.

8. Pour the batter into the baking dish and bake for about 1 hour or until a wooden pick inserted in the middle comes out clean.
9. Serve warm with a dusting of powdered sugar.

Nutrition:
- Calories: 232
- Fat: 5 g
- Carbohydrates: 42 g
- Phosphorus: 54 mg
- Potassium: 104 mg
- Sodium: 18 mg
- Protein: 4 g

353. Elegant Lavender Cookies
Preparation Time: 10 minutes
Cooking Time: 15 minutes
Servings: Makes 24 cookies
Ingredients:
- 5 dried organic lavender flowers, the entire top of the flower
- ½ cup granulated sugar
- 1 cup unsalted butter, at room temperature
- 2 cups all-purpose flour
- 1 cup rice flour

Directions:
1. Strip the tiny lavender flowers off the main stem carefully and place the flowers and granulated sugar into a food processor or blender. Pulse until the mixture is finely chopped.
2. In a medium bowl, cream together the butter and lavender sugar until it is very fluffy.
3. Mix the flours into the creamed mixture until the mixture resembles fine crumbs.
4. Gather the dough together into a ball and then roll it into a long log.
5. Wrap the cookie dough in plastic and refrigerate it for about 1 hour or until firm.
6. Preheat the oven to 375°F.
7. Slice the chilled dough into ¼-inch rounds and refrigerate it for 1 hour or until firm.
8. Bake the cookies for 15 to 18 minutes or until they are a very pale, golden brown.
9. Let the cookies cool.
10. Store the cookies at room temperature in a sealed container for up to 1 week.

Nutrition:
- Calories: 153
- Fat: 9 g
- Carbohydrates: 17 g
- Phosphorus: 18 mg
- Potassium: 17 mg
- Sodium: 0 mg
- Protein: 1 g

354. Carob Angel Food Cake
Preparation Time: 30 minutes
Cooking Time: 30 minutes
Servings: 16
Ingredients:
- ¾ cup all-purpose flour
- ¼ cup carob flour
- 1½ cups sugar, divided
- 12 large egg whites, at room temperature
- 1½ teaspoons cream of tartar
- 2 teaspoons vanilla

Directions:
1. Preheat the oven to 375°F.
2. In a medium bowl, sift together the all-purpose flour, carob flour, and ¾ cup of the sugar; set aside.
3. Beat the egg whites and cream of tartar with a hand mixer for about 5 minutes or until soft peaks form.
4. Add the remaining ¾ cup sugar by the tablespoon to the egg whites until all the sugar is used up and stiff peaks form.
5. Fold in the flour mixture and vanilla.
6. Spoon the batter into an angel food cake pan.
7. Run a knife through the batter to remove any air pockets.
8. Bake the cake for about 30 minutes or until the top springs back when pressed lightly.
9. Invert the pan onto a wire rack to cool.
10. Run a knife around the rim of the cake pan and remove the cake from the pan.

Nutrition:
- Calories: 113
- Fat: 0 g
- Carbohydrates: 25 g
- Phosphorus: 11 mg
- Potassium: 108 mg
- Sodium: 42 mg
- Protein: 3 g

355. Old-fashioned Apple Kuchen
Preparation Time: 25 minutes
Cooking Time: 1 hour
Servings: 16
Ingredients:
- Unsalted butter, for greasing the baking dish
- 1 cup unsalted butter, at room temperature
- 2 cups granulated sugar
- 2 eggs, beaten
- 2 teaspoons pure vanilla extract
- 2 cups all-purpose flour
- 1 teaspoon Ener-G baking soda substitute
- 2 teaspoons ground cinnamon
- ½ teaspoon ground nutmeg
- Pinch ground allspice
- 2 large apples, peeled, cored, and diced (about 3 cups)

Directions:
1. Preheat the oven to 350°F.
2. Grease a 9-by-13-inch glass baking dish; set aside.
3. Cream together the butter and sugar with a hand mixer until light and fluffy, for about 3 minutes.
4. Add the eggs and vanilla and beat until combined, scraping down the sides of the bowl, about 1 minute.
5. In a small bowl, stir together the flour, baking soda substitute, cinnamon, nutmeg, and allspice.
6. Add the dry ingredients to the wet ingredients and stir to combine.
7. Stir in the apple and spoon the batter into the baking dish.
8. Bake for about 1 hour or until the cake is golden.
9. Cool the cake on a wire rack.
10. Serve warm or chilled.

Nutrition:
- Calories: 368
- Fat: 16 g
- Carbohydrates: 53 g
- Phosphorus: 46 mg
- Potassium: 68 mg

- Sodium: 15 mg
- Protein: 3 g

356. Dessert Cocktail
Preparation Time: 1 minute
Cooking Time: 0 minutes
Servings: 4
Ingredients:
- 1 cup of cranberry juice
- 1 cup of fresh ripe strawberries, washed and hull removed
- 2 tablespoon of lime juice
- ¼ cup of white sugar
- 8 ice cubes

Directions:
1. Combine all the ingredients in a blender until smooth and creamy.
2. Pour the liquid into tall chilled glasses and serve cold.

Nutrition:
- Calories: 92
- Carbohydrate: 23.5 g
- Protein: 0.5 g
- Sodium: 3.62 mg
- Potassium: 103.78 mg
- Phosphorus: 17.86 mg
- Dietary Fiber: 0.84 g
- Fat: 0.17 g

357. Baked Egg Custard
Preparation Time: 15 minutes
Cooking Time: 30 minutes
Servings: 4
Ingredients:
- 2 medium eggs, at room temperature
- ¼ cup of semi-skimmed milk
- 3 tablespoons of white sugar
- ½ teaspoon of nutmeg
- 1 teaspoon of vanilla extract

Directions:
1. Preheat your oven at 375 F/180C
2. Mix all the ingredients in a mixing bowl and beat with a hand mixer for a few seconds until creamy and uniform.
3. Pour the mixture into lightly greased muffin tins.
4. Bake for 25-30 minutes or until the knife you place inside comes out clean.

Nutrition:
- Calories: 96.56
- Carbohydrate: 10.5 g
- Protein: 3.5 g
- Sodium: 37.75 mg
- Potassium: 58.19 mg
- Phosphorus: 58.76 mg
- Dietary Fiber: 0.06 g
- Fat: 2.91 g

358. Gumdrop Cookies
Preparation Time: 15 minutes
Cooking Time: 12 minutes
Servings: 25
Ingredients:
- ½ cup of spreadable unsalted butter
- 1 medium egg
- 1 cup of brown sugar
- 1 ⅔ cups of all-purpose flour, sifted
- ¼ cup of milk
- 1 teaspoon vanilla
- 1 teaspoon of baking powder
- 15 large gumdrops, chopped finely

Directions:
1. Preheat the oven at 400F/195C.
2. Combine the sugar, butter, and egg until creamy.
3. Add the milk and vanilla and stir well.

4. Combine the flour with the baking powder in a different bowl. Incorporate the sugar, butter mixture, and stir.
5. Add the gumdrops and place the mixture in the fridge for half an hour.
6. Drop the dough with tablespoonful into a lightly greased baking or cookie sheet.
7. Bake for 10-12 minutes or until golden brown.

Nutrition:
- Calories: 102.17
- Carbohydrate: 16.5 g
- Protein: 0.86 g
- Sodium: 23.42 mg
- Potassium: 45 mg
- Phosphorus: 32.15 mg
- Dietary Fiber: 0.13 g
- Fat: 4 g

359. Pound Cake with Pineapple
Preparation Time: 10 minutes
Cooking Time: 50 minutes
Servings: 24
Ingredients:
- 3 cups of all-purpose flour, sifted
- 3 cups of sugar
- 1 ½ cups of butter
- 6 whole eggs and 3 egg whites
- 1 teaspoon of vanilla extract
- 1 10-ounce can of pineapple chunks, rinsed and crushed (keep the juice aside).

For glaze:
- 1 cup of sugar
- 1 stick of unsalted butter or margarine
- Reserved juice from the pineapple

Directions:
1. Preheat the oven at 350F/180C.
2. Beat the sugar and the butter with a hand mixer until creamy and smooth.
3. Slowly add the eggs (one or two every time) and stir well after pouring each egg.
4. Add the vanilla extract, follow up with the flour and stir well.
5. Add the drained and chopped pineapple.
6. Pour the mixture into a greased cake tin and bake for 45-50 minutes.
7. In a small saucepan, combine the sugar with the butter and pineapple juice. Stir every few seconds and bring to boil. Cook until you get a creamy to thick glaze consistency.
8. Pour the glaze over the cake while still hot.
9. Let cook for at least 10 seconds and serve.

Nutrition:
- Calories: 407.4
- Carbohydrate: 79 g
- Protein: 4.25 g
- Sodium: 118.97 mg
- Potassium: 180.32 mg
- Phosphorus: 66.37 mg
- Dietary Fiber: 2.25 g
- Fat: 16.48 g

360. Apple Crunch Pie
Preparation Time: 10 minutes
Cooking Time: 35 minutes
Servings: 8
Ingredients
- 4 large tart apples, peeled, seeded and sliced
- ½ cup of white all-purpose flour
- ⅓ cup margarine
- 1 cup of sugar

- ¾ cup of rolled oat flakes
- ½ teaspoon of ground nutmeg

Directions
1. Preheat the oven to 375F/180C.
2. Place the apples over a lightly greased square pan (around 7 inches).
3. Mix the rest of the ingredients in a medium bowl and spread the batter over the apples.
4. Bake for 30-35 minutes or until the top crust has gotten golden brown.
5. Serve hot.

Nutrition:
- Calories: 261.9
- Carbohydrate: 47.2 g
- Protein: 1.5 g
- Sodium: 81 mg
- Potassium: 123.74 mg
- Phosphorus: 35.27 mg
- Dietary Fiber: 2.81 g
- Fat: 7.99 g

361. Vanilla Custard

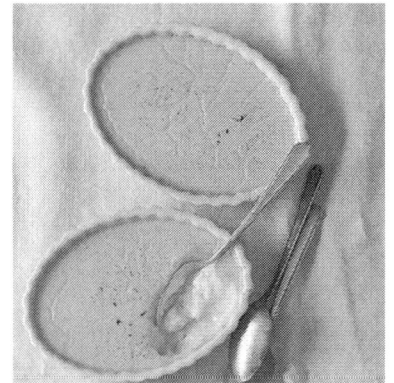

Preparation Time: 7 minutes
Cooking Time: 10 minutes
Servings: 10
Ingredients:
- 1 Egg
- 1/8 tsp Vanilla
- 1/8 tsp Nutmeg
- ½ cup Almond milk
- 2 Tbsp Stevia

Directions:
1. Scald the milk, then let it cool slightly.
2. Break the egg into a bowl and beat it with the nutmeg.
3. Add the scalded milk, the vanilla, and the sweetener to taste. Mix well.
4. Place the bowl in a baking pan filled with ½ deep of water.
5. Bake for 30 minutes at 325F.
6. Serve.

Nutrition:
- Calories: 167.3
- Fat: 9 g
- Carbs: 11 g
- Phosphorus: 205 mg
- Potassium: 249 mg
- Sodium: 124 mg
- Protein: 10 g

362. Chocolate Chip Cookies

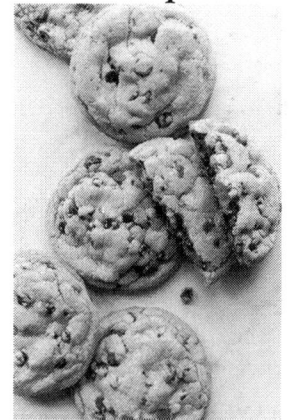

Preparation Time: 7 minutes
Cooking Time: 10 minutes
Servings: 10
Ingredients:
- ½ cup Semi-sweet chocolate chips
- ½ tsp. Baking soda
- ½ tsp. Vanilla

- 1 Egg
- 1 cup Flour
- ½ cup Margarine
- 4 tsp. Stevia

Directions:
1. Sift the dry ingredients.
2. Cream the margarine, stevia, vanilla, and egg with a whisk.
3. Add flour mixture and beat well.
4. Stir in the chocolate chips, then drop a teaspoonful of the mixture over a greased baking sheet.
5. Bake the cookies for about 10 minutes at 375F.
6. Cool and serve.

Nutrition:
- Calories: 106.2
- Fat: 7 g
- Carbs: 8. 9 g
- Phosphorus: 19 mg
- Potassium: 28 mg
- Sodium: 98 mg
- Protein: 1.5 g

363. Coconut Loaf

Preparation Time: 15 minutes
Cooking Time: 40 minutes
Servings: 4
Ingredients:
- 1 ½ tablespoons coconut flour
- ¼ teaspoon baking powder
- 1/8 teaspoon salt
- 1 tablespoon coconut oil, melted
- 1 whole egg

Directions:
1. Preheat your oven to 350 °F.
2. Add coconut flour, baking powder, salt.
3. Add coconut oil, eggs, and stir well until mixed.
4. Leave the batter for several minutes.
5. Pour half the batter onto the baking pan.
6. Spread it to form a circle, repeat with remaining batter.
7. Bake in the oven for 10 minutes.
8. Once a golden-brown texture comes, let it cool and serve.
9. Enjoy!

Nutrition:
- Calories: 297
- Fat: 14 g
- Carbohydrates: 15 g
- Protein: 15 g

364. Chocolate Parfait

Preparation Time: 2 hours
Cooking Time: nil
Servings: 4
Ingredients:
- 2 tablespoons cocoa powder
- 1 cup almond milk
- 1 tablespoon chia seeds
- Pinch of salt
- ½ teaspoon vanilla extract

Directions:
1. Take a bowl and add cocoa powder, almond milk, chia seeds, vanilla extract, and stir.
2. Transfer to dessert glass and place in your fridge for 2 hours.
3. Serve and enjoy!

Nutrition:
- Calories: 130
- Fat: 5 g
- Carbohydrates: 7 g
- Protein: 16 g

365. Cauliflower Bagel
Preparation Time: 10 minutes
Cooking Time: 30 minutes
Servings: 12
Ingredients:
- 1 large cauliflower, divided into florets and roughly chopped
- ¼ cup nutritional yeast
- ¼ cup almond flour
- ½ teaspoon garlic powder
- 1 ½ teaspoon fine sea salt
- 2 whole eggs
- 1 tablespoon sesame seeds

Directions:
1. Preheat your oven to 400 °F.
2. Line a baking sheet with parchment paper, keep it on the side.
3. Blend cauliflower in a food processor and transfer to a bowl.
4. Add nutritional yeast, almond flour, garlic powder, and salt to a bowl, mix
5. Take another bowl and whisk in eggs, add to cauliflower mix.
6. Give the dough a stir.
7. Incorporate the mixture into the egg mix.
8. Make balls from the dough, making a hole using your thumb into each ball.
9. Arrange them on your prepped sheet, flattening them into bagel shapes.
10. Sprinkle sesame seeds and bake for half an hour.
11. Remove the oven and let them cool, enjoy!

Nutrition:
- Calories: 152
- Fat: 10 g
- Carbohydrates: 4 g
- Protein: 4 g

366. Lemon Mousse
Preparation Time: 10 + chill time
Cooking Time: 10 minutes
Servings: 4
Ingredients:
- 1 cup coconut cream
- 8 ounces' cream cheese, soft
- ¼ cup fresh lemon juice
- 3 pinches salt
- 1 teaspoon lemon liquid stevia

Directions:
1. Preheat your oven to 350 °F.
2. Grease a ramekin with butter
3. Beat cream, cream cheese, fresh lemon juice, salt, and lemon liquid stevia in a mixer.
4. Pour batter into the ramekin.
5. Bake for 10 minutes, then transfer the mousse to a serving glass.
6. Let it chill for 2 hours and serve.
7. Enjoy!

Nutrition:
- Calories: 395
- Fat: 31 g
- Carbohydrates: 3 g
- Protein: 5 g

367. Jalapeno Crisp
Preparation Time: 10 minutes
Cooking Time: 1 hour 15 minutes
Servings: 20
Ingredients:
- 1 cup sesame seeds
- 1 cup sunflower seeds
- 1 cup flaxseeds
- ½ cup hulled hemp seeds
- 3 tablespoons Psyllium husk
- 1 teaspoon salt
- 1 teaspoon baking powder
- 2 cups of water

Directions:
1. Preheat your oven to 350 °F.
2. Take your blender and add seeds, baking powder, salt, and Psyllium husk.
3. Blend well until a sand-like texture appears.
4. Stir in water and mix until a batter forms.
5. Allow the batter to rest for 10 minutes until a dough-like thick mixture forms.
6. Pour the dough onto a cookie sheet lined with parchment paper.
7. Spread it evenly, making sure that it has a thickness of ¼ inch thick all around.
8. Bake for 75 minutes in your oven.
9. Remove and cut into 20 spices.
10. Allow them to cool for 30 minutes and enjoy!

Nutrition:
- Calories: 156
- Fat: 13 g
- Carbohydrates: 2 g
- Protein: 5 g

368. Raspberry Popsicle
Preparation Time: 2 hours
Cooking Time: 15 minutes
Servings: 4
Ingredients:
- 1 ½ cups raspberries
- 2 cups of water

Directions:
1. Take a pan and fill it up with water.
2. Add raspberries.
3. Place it over medium heat and bring to water to a boil.
4. Reduce the heat and simmer for 15 minutes.
5. Remove heat and pour the mix into Popsicle molds.
6. Add a popsicle stick and let it chill for 2 hours.
7. Serve and enjoy!

Nutrition:
- Calories: 58
- Fat: 0.4 g
- Carbohydrates: 0 g
- Protein: 1.4 g

369. Easy Fudge
Preparation Time: 15 minutes + chill time
Cooking Time: 5 minutes
Servings: 25
Ingredients:
- 1 ¾ cups of coconut butter
- 1 cup pumpkin puree
- 1 teaspoon ground cinnamon
- ¼ teaspoon ground nutmeg
- 1 tablespoon coconut oil

Directions:
1. Take an 8x8 inch square baking pan and line it with aluminum foil.
2. Take a spoon and scoop out the coconut butter into a heated pan and allow the butter to melt.
3. Keep stirring well and remove from the heat once fully melted.
4. Add spices and pumpkin and keep straining until you have a grain-like texture.
5. Add coconut oil and keep stirring to incorporate everything.
6. Scoop the mixture into your baking pan and evenly distribute it.
7. Place wax paper on top of the mixture and press gently to straighten the top.
8. Remove the paper and discard.
9. Allow it to chill for 1-2 hours.

10. Once chilled, take it out and slice it up into pieces.
11. Enjoy!

Nutrition:
- Calories: 120
- Fat: 10 g
- Carbohydrates: 5 g
- Protein: 1.2 g

370. Cashew and Almond Butter
Preparation Time: 5 minutes
Cooking Time: Nil
Servings: 1
Ingredients:
- 1 cup almonds, blanched
- 1/3 cup cashew nuts
- 2 tablespoons coconut oil
- Salt as needed
- ½ teaspoon cinnamon

Directions:
1. Preheat your oven to 350 °F.
2. Bake almonds and cashews for 12 minutes. Let them cool.
3. Transfer to a food processor and add remaining ingredients.
4. Add oil and keep blending until smooth.
5. Serve and enjoy!

Nutrition:
- Calories: 205 Fat: 19 g
- Carbohydrates: 0 g
- Protein: 2.8 g

371. Instant Pot Cheesecake
Preparation Time: 10 minutes
Cooking Time: 38 minutes
Servings: 4
Ingredients:
Graham Cracker Crust:
- 3 tablespoons sugar
- 5 tablespoons unsalted butter
- 9 large graham crackers, pulsed into crumbs
- 2 tablespoons ground pecans
- ¼ teaspoons cinnamon

Cheesecake Filling:
- 12 oz. cream cheese
- 2 teaspoons lemon zest
- 2 teaspoons vanilla extract
- 1 tablespoon cornstarch
- ½ cup + 2 tablespoons granulated sugar
- 2 large eggs + 1 egg yolk
- ½ cup sour cream

Directions:
1. Start by heating sugar with butter in the microwave for 40 seconds.
2. Blend this melt with the cinnamon, pecan, and crumbs in a food processor.
3. Spread this mixture at the bottom of a baking pan.
4. Place this crust in the freezer for 1 hour.
5. Meanwhile, prepare the filling by beating all of its ingredients in an electric mixer.
6. Spread this filling into the prepared crust evenly.
7. Pour 2 cups of water into the Instant Pot and place the steam rack over it.
8. Place the baking pan over the rack and seal the lid.
9. Select Manual mode with high pressure for 37 minutes.
10. Once the cooking is done, naturally release the pressure and remove the lid after 25 minutes.
11. Allow it to cool, then remove the pie from the pan.
12. Refrigerate for 3 hours at minimum.

13. Slice and serve.

Nutrition:
- Calories: 177
- Total Fats: 9 g
- Saturated Fat: 8.5 g
- Cholesterol: 21 mg
- Sodium: 95 mg
- Total Carbs: 21 g
- Fiber: 1.0 g
- Sugar: 2.3 g
- Protein: 3 g

372. Pots De Crème
Preparation Time: 10 minutes
Cooking Time: 6 minutes
Servings: 6
Ingredients:
- 1 ½ cups heavy cream
- ½ cup coconut milk
- 5 large egg yolks
- ¼ cup sugar
- 8 oz. bittersweet chocolate, melted
- Whipped cream and grated chocolate to garnish

Directions:
1. Start by heating cream with milk in a saucepan to a simmer.
2. Meanwhile, beat egg yolks with sugar in a bowl.
3. Slowly pour in the hot milk mixture whiles stirring continuously.
4. Add chocolate and mix until fully incorporated.
5. Divide this mixture into 6 custard cups of equal size.
6. Pour 1.5 cups water into the Instant Pot and place the double steam rack over it.
7. Place the 3 custard cups over one rack and the other 3 on the top rack.
8. Seal the pot's lid and cook for 6 minutes on "Manual" mode with High pressure.
9. Once the cooking is done, release the pressure completely, then remove the lid.
10. Refrigerate the cups for 4 hours or more.
11. Serve.

Nutrition:
- Calories: 204
- Total Fats: 8 g
- Saturated Fat: 5.1 g
- Cholesterol: 43 mg
- Sodium: 113 mg
- Total Carbs: 30 g
- Fiber: 0.5 g
- Sugar: 1.2 g
- Protein: 3 g

373. Ingredient Cheesecake
Preparation Time: 10 minutes
Cooking Time: 25 minutes
Servings: 4
Ingredients:
Date and Nut Crust:
- 1 cup nuts

Oatmeal Cookie Crust:
- ½ cup rolled oats
- ¼ cup pecans
- ¼ cup brown sugar
- 3 tablespoons melted butter

Ingredient Cheesecake:
- 1 (14 ounces) can coconut milk with cream
- 1 cup yogurt
- Oil or butter, for greasing ramekins or cheesecake pan

Directions:
1. Start by mixing the yogurt with the milk in a bowl.
2. Divide this mixture into 4 four ramekins, greased with cooking oil.
3. Place these ramekins in a baking pan.
4. After pouring 2 cups of water into the Instant Pot, place the steam rack over it.
5. Cover the ramekins with aluminum foil and place the baking pan over the rack.
6. Seal the pot's lid and cook for 25 minutes on Manual mode with high pressure.
7. Once the cooking is done, release the pressure completely, then remove the lid.
8. Allow the ramekins to cool at room temperature.
9. Refrigerate them for 6 hours.
10. Garnish as desired.

Nutrition:
- Calories: 258
- Total Fats: 13 g
- Saturated Fat: 9.1 g
- Cholesterol: 11 mg
- Sodium: 214 mg
- Total Carbs: 28 g
- Fiber: 1.0 g
- Sugar: 1.3 g
- Protein: 5 g

374. Egg Leche Flan

Preparation Time: 10 minutes
Cooking Time: 12 minutes
Servings: 4
Ingredients:
Caramel:
- ½ cup white sugar
- 2 tablespoons water

Custard:
- 4 large eggs
- 1 can (14 oz.) coconut cream milk
- 1 can (12 oz.) almond milk
- 1 teaspoon pure vanilla extract or lemon zest

Directions:
1. Start by mixing sugar with water in a bowl, then heat for 4 minutes in the microwave.
2. Mix well, then divide this mixture into a baking dish.
3. Now whisk eggs with milk, lemon zest, vanilla, and coconut milk in a bowl.
4. Pour this mixture into the baking dish.
5. After pouring 1.5 cups of water into the Instant pot, place a steam rack over it.
6. Place the baking dish over the rack and seal the pot's lid.
7. Cook for 12 minutes on Manual mode with high pressure.
8. Once the cooking is done, release the pressure completely, then remove the pot's lid.
9. Allow the flan to cool down, then refrigerate for 3 hours.

Nutrition:
- Calories: 150
- Total Fats: 6 g
- Saturated Fat: 1.5 g
- Cholesterol: 24 mg
- Sodium: 67 mg
- Total Carbs: 22 g
- Fiber: 0.2 g
- Sugar: 2.4 g
- Protein: 2 g

375. Pot Chocolate Pudding Cake

Preparation Time: 10 minutes
Cooking Time: 4 minutes
Servings: 4
Ingredients:

- 2/3 cup chopped dark chocolate
- ½ cup applesauce
- 2 eggs
- 1 teaspoon vanilla
- ¼ cup arrowroot
- 3 tablespoons cocoa powder
- Powdered sugar for topping

Directions:
1. Start by pouring 2 cups of water into the Instant pot and place trivet over it.
2. Add chocolate to a ramekin and place it over the trivet.
3. Switch the Instant pot to the Sauté mode and cook until the chocolate melts.
4. Whisk eggs, applesauce, and vanilla in a mixing bowl.
5. Stir in all the dry ingredients and mix well until fully incorporated.
6. Grease a 6-inch pan with butter and dust it with flour.
7. Spread the batter in the pan and place it in the Instant Pot.
8. Seal the lid and cook for 4 minutes on Manual mode with High Pressure.
9. Once the cooking is done, release the pressure completely, then remove the pot's lid.
10. Allow the cake to cool, then remove it from the pan.

Nutrition:

- Calories: 210
- Total Fats: 7 g
- Saturated Fat: 4.5 g
- Cholesterol: 23 mg
- Sodium: 58 mg
- Total Carbs: 35 g
- Fiber: 1.0 g
- Sugar: 2.9 g
- Protein: 2 g

376. Carrot Cake

Preparation Time: 10 minutes
Cooking Time: 50 minutes
Servings: 4
Ingredients:
Dry Cake Ingredients:

- 1 ½ cups whole wheat pastry flour
- 3/4 teaspoons baking powder
- 3/4 teaspoons baking soda
- ½ teaspoons ground cinnamon
- ¼ teaspoons ground cardamom
- ¼ teaspoons ground allspice
- ¼ teaspoons ground ginger

Wet Cake Ingredients:

- 2 tablespoons ground flaxseed, mixed with ¼ cup warm water
- ½ cup almond milk
- ½ teaspoons orange flower water, or substitute vanilla

Cake Mix in Ingredients:

- 1 cup shredded carrot

Icing Ingredients:

- ½ cup cashews
- ½ cup water, plus more as needed
- 1 ½ teaspoons orange flower water

Directions:
1. Start by adding 1.5 cups of water into Instant Pot and place a trivet over it.
2. Grease a pan with cooking oil, suitable to fit the Instant Pot.
3. Prepare the batter by mixing the dry and wet ingredients separately.

4. Now mix the two mixtures in a large bowl.
5. Spread this batter in the prepared, and then cover it with aluminum foil.
6. Place the pan in the Instant Pot and seal its lid.
7. Cook for 50 minutes on "Manual" mode with high pressure.
8. Meanwhile, prepare the icing by cooking cashews, date, and water in a saucepan to boil.
9. Allow it to cool, then blend this mixture in a blender until smooth.
10. Spread this icing over the baked cake.

Nutrition:
- Calories: 184
- Total Fats: 9 g
- Saturated Fat: 4.5 g
- Cholesterol: 0 mg
- Sodium: 94 mg
- Total Carbs: 22 g
- Fiber: 8 g
- Sugar: 0.8 g
- Protein: 4 g

377. Pumpkin Chocolate Cake
Preparation Time: 10 minutes
Cooking Time: 20 minutes
Servings: 6
Ingredients:
- 2 cups flour
- 1 tablespoon pumpkin pie spice
- 1 teaspoon baking soda
- 2 sticks- 1 cup unsalted butter, softened
- 1-¼ cup sugar
- 1 egg
- 2 teaspoons vanilla extract
- 1 cup cream cheese
- 1 package 12 oz. chocolate chips

Directions:
1. Whisk pumpkin pie spice, flour, and baking soda in a mixing bowl.
2. Beat sugar with butter in a mixer until fluffy.
3. Whisk in egg, vanilla, and cream cheese.
4. Beat well, then gradually add the flour mixture while mixing continuously.
5. Fold in the chocolate chips and grease 2 Bundt pans with cooking oil.
6. Divide the batter into the pans and cover them with aluminum foil.
7. Pour 1.5 cups of water into the Instant Pot and place rack over it.
8. Set one Bundt on the rack and seal the lid.
9. Cook for 20 minutes on Manual mode with High pressure.
10. Once done, release the pressure completely, then remove the lid.
11. Cook the other cake in the Bundt pan following the same method.
12. Allow the cakes to cool, then slice to serve.

Nutrition:
- Calories: 232 Total Fats: 11 g
- Saturated Fat: 6.5 g
- Cholesterol: 7 mg
- Sodium: 112 mg
- Total Carbs: 30 g
- Fiber: 0.4 g Sugar: 0.5 g
- Protein: 3 g

378. Apple Pie
Preparation Time: 10 minutes
Cooking Time: 50 minutes
Servings: 6
Ingredients:
- 6 medium apples, peeled, cored & sliced

- ½ cup granulated sugar
- 1 tsp ground cinnamon
- 6 tbsp butter
- 2-2/3 cups all-purpose flour
- 1 cup shortening
- 6 tbsp water

Directions:
1. Preheat your oven to 425 degrees F.
2. Toss the apple slices with cinnamon and sugar in a bowl and set it aside covered.
3. Blend the flour with the shortening in a pastry blender, then add chilled water by the tablespoon.
4. Continue mixing and adding the water until it forms a smooth dough ball.
5. Divide the dough into two equal-size pieces and spread them into 2 separate 9-inch sheets.
6. Arrange the sheet of dough at the bottom of a 9-inch pie pan.
7. Spread the apples in the pie shell and spread a tablespoon of butter over it.
8. Cover the filling with the remaining sheet of the dough and pinch down the edges.
9. Carve 1-inch cuts on top of the pie and bake for 50 minutes or more until golden.
10. Slice and serve.

Nutrition:
- Calories: 517 Protein: 4 g
- Carbohydrates: 51 g
- Fat: 33 g
- Cholesterol: 24 mg
- Sodium: 65 mg
- Potassium: 145 mg
- Phosphorus: 43 mg
- Calcium: 24 mg
- Fiber: 2.7 g

379. Blueberry Cream Cones

Preparation Time: 10 minutes
Cooking Time: 0 minutes
Servings: 6
Ingredients:
- 4 oz cream cheese
- 1-½ cup whipped topping
- 1-¼ cup fresh or frozen blueberries
- ¼ cup blueberry jam or preserves
- 6 small ice cream cones

Directions:
1. Start by softening the cream cheese, then beat it in a mixer until fluffy.
2. Fold in jam and fruits.
3. Divide the mixture into the ice cream cones.
4. Serve fresh.

Nutrition:
- Calories: 177
- Protein: 3 g
- Carbohydrates: 21 g
- Fat: 9 g
- Cholesterol: 21 mg
- Sodium: 95 mg
- Potassium: 81 mg
- Phosphorus: 40 mg
- Calcium: 24 mg
- Fiber: 1.0 g

380. Cherry Coffee Cake

Preparation Time: 10 minutes
Cooking Time: 40 minutes
Total Time: 50 minutes
Servings: 6
Ingredients:
- ½ cup unsalted butter
- 2 eggs
- 1 cup granulated sugar
- 1 cup sour cream

- 1 tsp vanilla
- 2 cups all-purpose white flour
- 1 tsp baking powder
- 1 tsp baking soda
- 20 oz cherry pie filling

Directions:
1. Preheat oven to 350 degrees F.
2. Soften the butter, first then beat it with the eggs, sugar, vanilla, and sour cream in a mixer.
3. Separately mix flour with baking soda and baking powder.
4. Add this mixture to the egg mixture and mix well until smooth.
5. Spread this batter evenly in a 9x13 inch baking pan.
6. Bake the pie for 40 minutes in the oven until golden on the surface.
7. Slice and serve with cherry pie filling on top.

Nutrition:
- Calories: 204
- Protein: 3 g
- Carbohydrates: 30 g
- Fat: 8 g
- Cholesterol: 43 mg
- Sodium: 113 mg
- Potassium: 72 mg
- Phosphorus: 70 mg
- Calcium: 41 mg
- Fiber: 0.5 g

381. Cherry Dessert
Preparation Time: 10 minutes
Cooking Time: 20 minutes
Total Time: 30 minutes
Servings: 6
Ingredients:
- 1 small package sugar-free cherry gelatin
- 1 pie crust, 9-inch size
- 8 oz light cream cheese
- 12 oz whipped topping
- 20 oz cherry pie filling

Directions:
1. Prepare the cherry gelatin as per the given instructions on the packet.
2. Pour the mixture into an 8x8 inch pan and refrigerate until set.
3. Soften the cream cheese at room temperature.
4. Place the 9-inch pie crust in a pie pan and bake it until golden brown.
5. Vigorously, beat the cream cheese in a mixer until fluffy and fold in whipped topping.
6. Dice the gelatin into cubes and add them to the cream cheese mixture.
7. Mix gently, then add this mixture to the baking pie shell.
8. Top the cream cheese filling with cherry pie filling.
9. Refrigerate for 3 hours, then slice to serve.

Nutrition:
- Calories: 258 Protein: 5 g
- Carbohydrates: 28 g Fat: 13 g
- Cholesterol: 11 mg
- Sodium: 214 mg
- Potassium: 150 mg
- Phosphorus: 50 mg
- Calcium: 30 mg Fiber: 1.0 g

382. Crunchy Peppermint Cookies
Preparation Time: 10 minutes
Cooking Time: 12 minutes
Total time: 22 minutes
Servings: 6
Ingredients:
- ½ cup unsalted butter

- 18 peppermint candies
- 3/4 cup sugar
- 1 large egg
- ¼ tsp peppermint extract
- 1-½ cups all-purpose flour
- 1 tsp baking powder

Directions:
1. Soften the butter at room temperature.
2. Add 12 peppermint candies to a zip lock bag and crush them using a mallet.
3. Beat butter with egg, sugar, and peppermint extract in a mixer until fluffy.
4. Stir in baking powder and flour and mix well until smooth.
5. Stir in crushed peppermint candies and refrigerate the dough for 1 hour.
6. Meanwhile, layer a baking sheet with parchment paper.
7. Preheat the oven to 350 degrees F.
8. Crush the remaining candies and keep them aside.
9. Make ¾-inch balls out of the dough and place them on the baking sheet.
10. Sprinkle the crushed candies over the balls.
11. Bake them for 12 minutes until slightly browned.
12. Serve fresh and enjoy.

Nutrition:
- Calories: 150 Protein: 2 g
- Carbohydrates: 22 g Fat: 6 g
- Cholesterol: 24 mg
- Sodium: 67 mg
- Potassium: 17 mg
- Phosphorus: 24 mg
- Calcium: 20 mg
- Fiber: 0.2 g

383. Cranberries Snow
Preparation Time: 10 minutes
Cooking Time: 12 minutes
Servings: 4
Ingredients:
- 1 cup cran-cherry juice
- 12 oz fresh cranberries
- 2 packets gelatin
- 2 cups granulated sugar
- 1 cup crushed pineapple
- 8 oz cream cheese
- 3 cups whipped topping

Directions:
1. Boil the cran-cherry juice in a saucepan.
2. Stir in cranberries and cook for 12 minutes.
3. Remove the pan from the stove heat and add 1 ¼ cup sugar and gelatin.
4. Mix well until dissolved, then allow it to cool for 30 minutes.
5. Toss in drained pineapple and mix well, then pour it all into a 9x13 inch pan.
6. Refrigerate this mixture for 1 hour.
7. Prepare the snow topping by mixing the ¾ sugar and cream cheese in a mixer.
8. Spread this mixture over the refrigerated cranberry mixture.
9. Serve fresh.

Nutrition:
- Calories 210 Protein: 2 g
- Carbohydrates: 35 g Fat: 7 g
- Cholesterol: 23 mg
- Sodium: 58 mg
- Potassium: 65 mg
- Phosphorus: 25 mg
- Calcium: 28 mg
- Fiber: 1.0 g

384. Chia Pudding with Berries

Preparation Time: 10 minutes
Cooking Time: 0 minutes
Servings: 4
Ingredients:
- 2 cups vanilla almond milk, sweetened
- ½ cup chia seeds
- ¼ cup shredded sweetened coconut
- ¼ cup fresh blueberries
- 4 large strawberries

Directions:
1. Blend the almond milk with chia seeds in a blender.
2. Divide this mixture into the serving bowls.
3. Refrigerate them for 1 hour, then top them with a strawberry, blueberries, and coconut shreds.
4. Serve fresh.

Nutrition:
- Calories: 184
- Protein: 4 g
- Carbohydrates: 22 g
- Fat: 9 g
- Cholesterol: 0 mg
- Sodium: 94 mg
- Potassium: 199 mg
- Phosphorus: 200 mg
- Calcium: 362 mg
- Fiber: 8 g

385. Vanilla Delight

Preparation Time: 10 minutes
Cooking Time: 25 minutes
Servings: 15
Ingredients:
- 1 cup all-purpose white flour
- 1 stick unsalted margarine
- 8 oz light cream cheese
- 8 oz whipped topping
- 1 cup granulated sugar
- 4 cartons vanilla pudding
- 1 tsp vanilla extract
- ½ cup shredded coconut, sweetened

Directions:
1. Preheat oven to 350 degrees F.
2. Mix the flour with margarine, then spread it in a 9x13 inch pan.
3. Bake this crust for 25 minutes until golden brown, then allow it to cool.
4. Beat the cream cheese with half of the whipped topping and sugar in a mixer.
5. Spread this mixture in the baked crust.
6. Mix pudding with vanilla extract in a separate bowl.
7. Spread the mixture over the cream cheese filling.
8. Garnish with the other half of the whipped topping.
9. Sprinkle coconut on top and refrigerate for 30 minutes.
10. Slice and serve.

Nutrition:
- Calories: 232 Protein: 3 g
- Carbohydrates: 30 g
- Fat: 11 g
- Cholesterol: 7 mg
- Sodium: 112 mg
- Potassium: 58 mg
- Phosphorus: 40 mg
- Calcium: 101 mg
- Fiber: 0.4 g

386. Chocolate Beet Cake

Preparation Time: 20 minutes
Cooking Time: 40 minutes
Servings: 12
Ingredients:
- 3 cups grated beets

- ¼ cup canola oil
- 4 eggs
- 4 oz. unsweetened chocolate
- 2 tsp. Phosphorus-free baking powder
- 2 cups all-purpose flour
- 1 cup sugar

Directions:
1. Set your oven to 325 F. Grease two 8-inch cake pans.
2. Mix the baking powder, flour, and sugar. Set aside.
3. Chop up the chocolate as finely as you can and melt using a double boiler. A microwave can also be used, but don't let it burn.
4. Allow it to cool, and then mix in the oil and eggs.
5. Mix all of the wet ingredients into the flour mixture and combine everything until well mixed.
6. Fold the beets in and pour the batter into the cake pans.
7. Let them bake for 40 to 50 minutes. To know it's done, the toothpick should come out clean when inserted into the cake.
8. Remove from the oven and allow them to cool.
9. Once cool, invert over a plate to remove.
10. This is great when served with whipped cream and fresh berries. Enjoy!

Nutrition:
- Calories: 270
- Protein: 6 g
- Sodium: 109 mg
- Potassium: 299 mg
- Phosphorus: 111 mg

387. Strawberry Pie
Preparation Time: 20 minutes
Cooking Time: 3 hours
Servings: 8
Ingredients:
For the crust:
- 1 ½ cups Graham cracker crumbs
- 5 tbsp. unsalted butter, at room temperature
- 2 tbsp. sugar

For the pie:
- 1 ½ tsp. gelatin powder
- 3 tbsp. cornstarch
- 3/4 cup sugar
- 5 cups sliced strawberries, divided
- 1 cup water

Directions:
For the crust:
1. Heat your oven to 375 F. Grease a pie pan.
2. Combine the butter, crumbs, and sugar and then press them into your pie pan.
3. Bake the crust for 10 to 15 minutes, until lightly browned.
4. Take out of the oven and let it cool completely.

For the pie:
1. Crush up a cup of strawberries.
2. Using a small pot, combine the sugar, water, gelatin, and cornstarch.
3. Bring the mixture in the pot up to a boil, lower the heat, and simmer until it has thickened.
4. Add in the crushed strawberries in the pot and let it simmer for another 5 minutes until the sauce has thickened up again.
5. Set it off the heat and pour it into a bowl.

6. Cool until it comes to room temperature.
7. Toss the remaining berries with the sauce to be well distributed and pour into the pie crust, and spread it out into an even layer.
8. Refrigerate the pie until cold. This will take about 3 hours. Serve and enjoy!

Nutrition:
- Calories: 265
- Protein: 3 g
- Sodium: 143 mg
- Potassium: 183 mg
- Phosphorus: 44 mg

388. Grape Skillet Galette
Preparation Time: 50 minutes
Cooking Time: 2 hours
Servings: 6
Ingredients:
For the Crust:
- ½ cup unsweetened rice milk
- 4 tbsp. cold butter
- 1 tbsp. sugar
- 1 cup all-purpose flour

For the Galette:
- 1 tbsp. cornstarch
- 1/3 cup sugar
- 1 egg white
- 2 cups halved seedless grapes

Directions:
For the crust:
1. Add the sugar and the flour to a food processor and mix for a few seconds.
2. Place in the butter and pulse until it looks like a coarse meal.
3. Add in the rice milk and combine until the dough forms.
4. Place the dough on a clean surface and shape it into a disc.
5. Wrap it with plastic wrap and place it in the fridge for 2 hours.

For the galette:
1. Set your oven to 425 F.
2. Mix the cornstarch and sugar and toss the grapes in.
3. Unwrap the dough and roll out on a floured surface.
4. Press it into a 14-inch circle and place it in a cast-iron skillet.
5. Add the grape filling in the center and spread out to fill, leaving a 2-inch crust. Fold the edge over.
6. Brush the crust with egg white and cook for 20 to 25 minutes. The crust should be golden.
7. Allow resting for 20 minutes before you serve. Enjoy!

Nutrition:
- Calories: 172
- Protein: 2 g
- Sodium: 65 mg
- Potassium: 69 mg
- Phosphorus: 21 mg

389. Small Chocolate Cakes
Preparation Time: 50 minutes
Cooking Time: 2 hours
Servings: 2
Ingredients:
- 1 box angel food cake mix
- 1 box lemon cake mix
- Water
- Nonstick cooking spray or batter
- Dark chocolate small squared chops and chocolate powder

Directions:
1. Use a transparent kitchen cooking bag and put it inside both lemon cake mix, angel food mix, and chocolate chips.

2. Mix everything and add water to prepare a small cupcake.
3. Put the mix in a mold to prepare a cupcake containing the ingredients and put in the microwave for one minute at a high temperature.
4. Slip the cupcake out of the mold and put it on a dish, let it cool, and put some more chocolate crumbs on it. Serve and enjoy!

Nutrition:
- Calories: 95
- Protein: 1 g
- Sodium: 162 mg
- Potassium: 15 mg
- Phosphorus: 80 mg

390. Strawberry Whipped Cream Cake

Preparation Time: 1 minute
Cooking Time: 30 minutes
Servings: 2
Ingredients:
- 1 pint whipping cream
- 2 tbsp. gelatin
- ½ glass cold water
- 1 glass boiling water
- 3 tbsp. lemon juice
- 1 orange glass juice
- 1 orange glass juice
- 1 tsp. sugar
- 3/4 cup sliced strawberries
- 1 large angel food cake or light sponge cake

Directions:
1. Put the gelatin in cold water, then add hot water and blend. Add orange and lemon juice, also add some sugar and go on blending.
2. Refrigerate and leave it there until you see it is starting to gel.
3. Whip half a portion of cream, add it to the mixture, strawberries, put wax paper in the bowl, and cut the cake into small pieces.
4. In between the pieces, add the whipped cream and put everything in the fridge for one night.
5. When you take out the cake, add some whipped cream on top and decorate some more fruit. Serve and enjoy!

Nutrition:
- Calories: 355
- Protein: 4 g
- Sodium: 275 mg
- Potassium: 145 mg
- Phosphorus: 145 mg

391. Sweet Cracker Pie Crust

Preparation Time: 15 minutes
Cooking Time: 30 minutes
Servings: 2
Ingredients:
- 1 bowl gelatin cracker crumbs
- ¼ small cup sugar
- Unsalted butter

Direction
1. Mix sweet cracker crumbs, butter, and sugar.
2. Put in the oven, preheat at 375°F.
3. Bake for 7 minutes, putting it in a greased pie.
4. Let the pie cool before adding any kind of filling. Serve and enjoy!

Nutrition:
- Calories: 205 Protein: 2 g
- Sodium: 208 mg
- Potassium: 67 mg
- Phosphorus: 22 mg

392. Apple Oatmeal Crunchy

Preparation Time: 20 minutes
Cooking Time: 20 minutes
Servings: 2
Ingredients:
- 5 green apples
- 1 bowl oatmeal
- A small cup brown sugar
- ½ cup flour
- 1 tsp. cinnamon
- ½ bowl butter

Direction
1. Prepare apples by cutting them into tiny slices and preheat the oven at 350°F.
2. In a cup mix oatmeal, flour, cinnamon and brown sugar.
3. Put butter in the batter and place sliced apple in a baking pan (9" x 13").
4. Spread oatmeal mixture over the apples and bake for 35 minutes. Serve and enjoy!

Nutrition:
- Calories: 295
- Protein: 3 g
- Sodium: 95 mg
- Potassium: 190 mg
- Phosphorus: 73 mg

393. Berry Ice Cream

Preparation Time: 25 minutes
Cooking Time: 30 minutes
Servings: 2
Ingredients:
- 6 ice cream cones
- 1 cup whipped topping
- 1 cup fresh blueberries
- 4 oz. cream cheese
- ¼ cup blueberry jam

Directions:
1. Put the cream cheese in a large cup and beat it with a mixer until it is fluffy.
2. Mix with fruit and jam and whipped topping.
3. Put the mixture on the small ice cream cones and refrigerate them in the freezer for 1 hour or more until they are ready to serve. Enjoy!

Nutrition:
- Calories: 175
- Protein: 3 g
- Sodium: 95 mg
- Potassium: 80 mg
- Phosphorus: 40 mg

394. Deliciously Good Scones

Preparation Time: 15 minutes
Cooking Time: 12 minutes
Servings: 10
Ingredients:
- 1/4 cup dried cranberries
- 1/4 cup sunflower seeds
- 1/2 teaspoon baking soda
- 1 large egg
- 2 cups all-purpose flour
- 2 tablespoon honey

Directions:
1. Preheat the oven to 3500F.
2. Grease a baking sheet. Set aside.
3. In a bowl, mix the salt, baking soda and flour. Add the dried fruits, nuts and seeds. Set aside.
4. In another bowl, mix the honey and eggs.
5. Add the wet ingredients to the dry ingredients. Use your hands to mix the dough.

6. Create 10 small round dough and place them on the baking sheet.
7. Bake for 12 minutes.

Nutrition:
- Calories: 44
- Carbs: 27 g
- Protein: 4 g
- Fat: 3 g
- Phosphorus: 59 mg
- Potassium: 92 mg
- Sodium: 65 mg

395. Mixed Berry Cobbler

Preparation Time: 15 minutes
Cooking Time: 4 hours
Servings: 8
Ingredients:
- 1/4 cup coconut milk
- 1/4 cup ghee
- 1/4 cup honey
- 1/2 cup almond flour
- 1/2 cup tapioca starch
- 1/2 tablespoon cinnamon
- 1/2 tablespoon coconut sugar
- 1 teaspoon vanilla
- 12 ounces frozen raspberries
- 16 ounces frozen wild blueberries
- 2 teaspoon baking powder
- 2 teaspoon tapioca starch

Directions:
1. Place the frozen berries in the slow cooker. Add honey and 2 teaspoons of tapioca starch. Mix to combine.
2. In a bowl, mix the tapioca starch, almond flour, coconut milk, ghee, baking powder and vanilla. Sweeten with sugar. Place this pastry mix on top of the berries.
3. Set the slow cooker for 4 hours.

Nutrition:
- Calories: 146
- Carbs: 33 g
- Protein: 1 g
- Fat: 3 g
- Phosphorus: 29 mg
- Potassium: 133 mg
- Sodium: 4 mg

396. Blueberry Espresso Brownies

Preparation Time: 15 minutes
Cooking Time: 30 minutes
Servings: 12
Ingredients:
- 1/4 cup organic cocoa powder
- 1/4 teaspoon salt
- 1/2 cup raw honey
- 1/2 teaspoon baking soda
- 1 cup blueberries
- 1 cup coconut cream
- 1 tablespoon cinnamon
- 1 tablespoon ground coffee
- 2 teaspoon vanilla extract
- 3 eggs

Directions:
1. Preheat the oven to 3250F.
2. In a bow mix together coconut cream, honey, eggs, cinnamon, honey, vanilla, baking soda, coffee and salt.
3. Use a mixer to combine all ingredients.
4. Fold in the blueberries.
5. Pour the batter in a greased baking dish and bake for 30 minutes or until a toothpick

inserted in the middle comes out clean.
6. Remove from the oven and let it cool.

Nutrition:
- Calories: 168
- Carbs: 20 g
- Protein: 4 g
- Fat: 10 g
- Phosphorus: 79 mg
- Potassium: 169 mg
- Sodium: 129 mg

397. Coffee Brownies
Preparation Time: 15 minutes
Cooking Time: 20 minutes
Servings: 4
Ingredients:
- 3 eggs, beaten
- 2 tablespoons cocoa powder
- 2 teaspoons Erythritol
- 1/2 cup almond flour
- 1/2 cup organic almond milk

Directions:
1. Place the eggs in the mixing bowl and combine them with Erythritol and almond milk.
2. With the help of the hand mixer, whisk the liquid until homogenous.
3. Then add almond flour and cocoa powder.
4. Whisk the mixture until smooth.
5. Take the non-sticky brownie mold and transfer the cocoa mass inside it.
6. Flatten it gently with the help of the spatula. The flattened mass should be thin.
7. Preheat the oven to 365F.
8. Transfer the brownie in the oven and bake it for 20 minutes.
9. Then chill the cooked brownies at least till the room temperature and cut into serving bars.

Nutrition:
- Calories: 78
- Fat: 5.8 g
- Fiber: 1.3 g
- Carbs: 2.7 g
- Protein: 5.5 g

398. Keto Marshmellow
Preparation Time: 15 minutes
Cooking Time: 5 minutes
Servings: 7
Ingredients:
- 1/4 cup water, boiled
- 4 tablespoons Erythritol
- 2 tablespoons gelatin powder
- 1 fl. oz. water

Directions:
1. Line the baking tray with the baking paper.
2. Pour 1 floozy of water in the shallow bowl and add gelatin. Stir it. Leave the gelatin.
3. Pour a 1/4 cup of water in the saucepan and bring it to boil.
4. Then add Erythritol and stir.
5. Bring the liquid to boil and keep cooking for 3 minutes over the medium-low heat.
6. Then switch off the heat.
7. Start to add gelatin mixture in the sweet water. Whisk it with the help of the hand mixer. Use the maximum speed.
8. When the mixture changes the color into white, whisk it for 1-2

minutes more or until you get strong peaks.
9. Very fast transfer the whisked mixture in the tray and flatten it.
10. Leave the marshmallow for 20 minutes to stabilize.
11. Then make the sharp knife wet and cut the marshmallow into cubes.

Nutrition:
- Calories: 7 Fat: 0 g
- Fiber: 0 g Carbs: 6.9 g Protein: 1.7 g

Conclusion

The kidneys are two bean-shaped organs that we all know about in passing. However, they are still greatly underappreciated. While people may know that they are a set of two organs that are a part of the urinary tract, too few people appreciate and understand their vital importance. Not only do kidneys help in the production of urine, but they also filter waste and toxins from our blood, remove these particles from our bodies, manage fluid and mineral levels, and synthesize vitamin D so that it can be utilized by our cells. With all of our kidneys' abilities, people are in a dangerous state when they have chronic kidney disease. Not only does this disease cause a person's kidney disease functioning to lessen, but it also can lead to kidney failure. When a person develops kidney failure, they cannot survive without either transplantation or blood dialysis treatments multiple times a week.

Thankfully, there is an option. The renal diet treats kidney disease and treats diabetes, and high blood pressure, allowing a person to stop the spread of kidney damage frequently. The purpose of this is to prevent kidney failure before it happens hopefully, and if a person does develop kidney failure, to then manage the condition along with other necessary treatments.

Making healthy food choices ensures that you are on the right track to take good care of your kidney health. The recipes included are packed with wholesome foods that provide your body with the necessary nutrients, including protein, healthy carbohydrates, and useful fats. I am sure this will serve its purpose to inspire my readers to understand and strictly follow the ideal renal diet to stay healthy and live the better lives they deserve.

Sodium, potassium, phosphorus, and proteins remain essential kidney-impacting nutrients to watch out for in a renal diet. As such, in line with the health-conscious objectives of this, several recipes are included along with their nutritional value. You need to ensure that you know what you are putting inside your body at all times.

It is strongly recommended that people with renal impairment strictly follow a renal or renal diet to reduce toxic compounds or waste in the bloodstream drastically. Toxic compounds, or rather, wastes in the blood, as many people call it, usually come from the type of food and liquids consumed. If a kidney is compromised or not functioning optimally, it simply means that the kidneys will not filter or dispose of waste as they should. If a toxic substance is not removed or left in the bloodstream, it is very harmful because it can negatively affect the patient's electrolyte level. Strict adherence to a renal diet greatly improves renal function and reduces the kidney's tendency to develop complete renal failure.

Printed in Great Britain
by Amazon